the *herbal* medicine chest

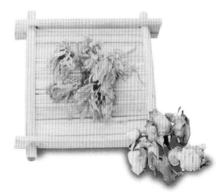

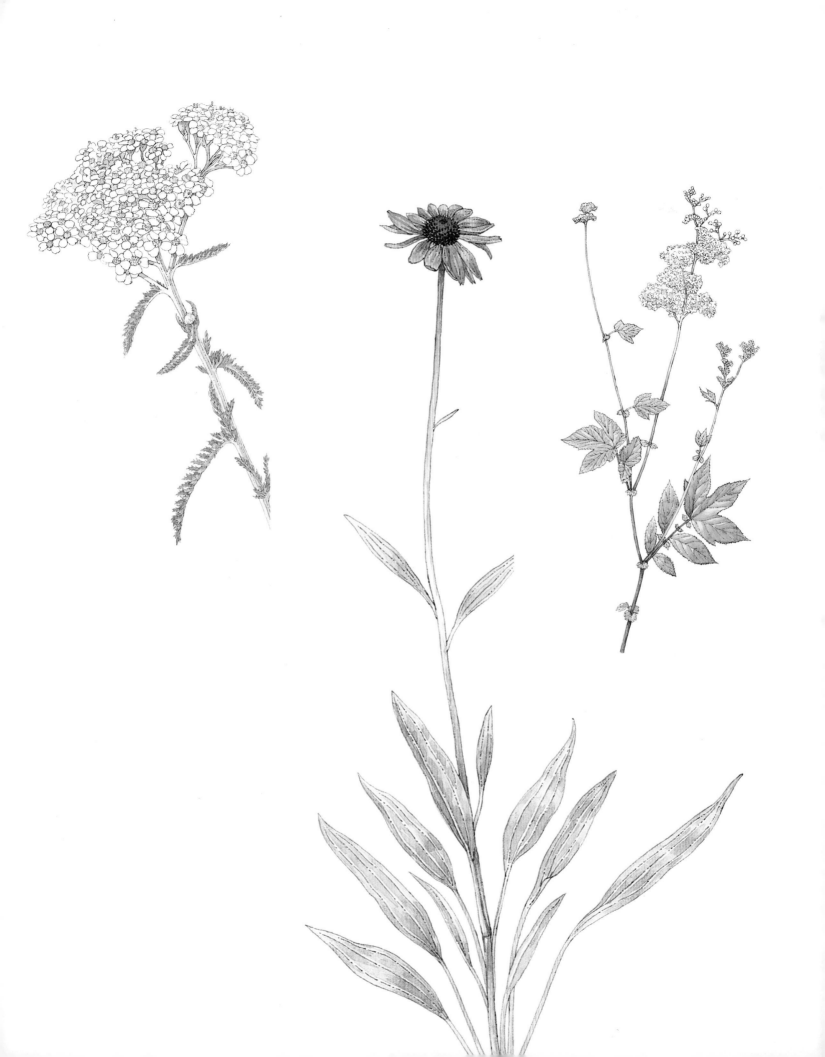

the *herbal* medicine chest

Sujata Bristow

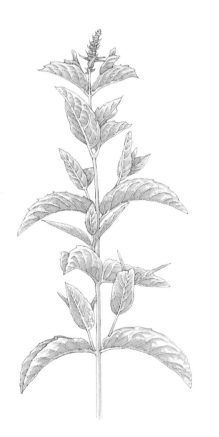

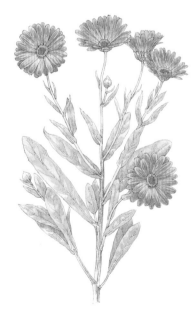

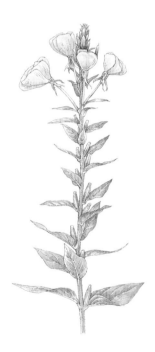

GRAMERCY
New York

This 2002 edition is published by Gramercy Books™, an imprint of Random House Value Publishing, 280 Park Avenue, New York, NY 10017, by arrangement with D&S Books, Cottage Meadow, Bocombe, Parkham, Bideford, Devon, England, EX39 5PH.

Gramercy is a registered trademark and the colophon is a trademark of Random House, Inc.

Printed in China

Random House
New York • Toronto • London • Sydney • Auckland

A catalog record for this title is available from the Library of Congress

ISBN: 0-517-16402-7

987654321

Contents

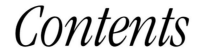

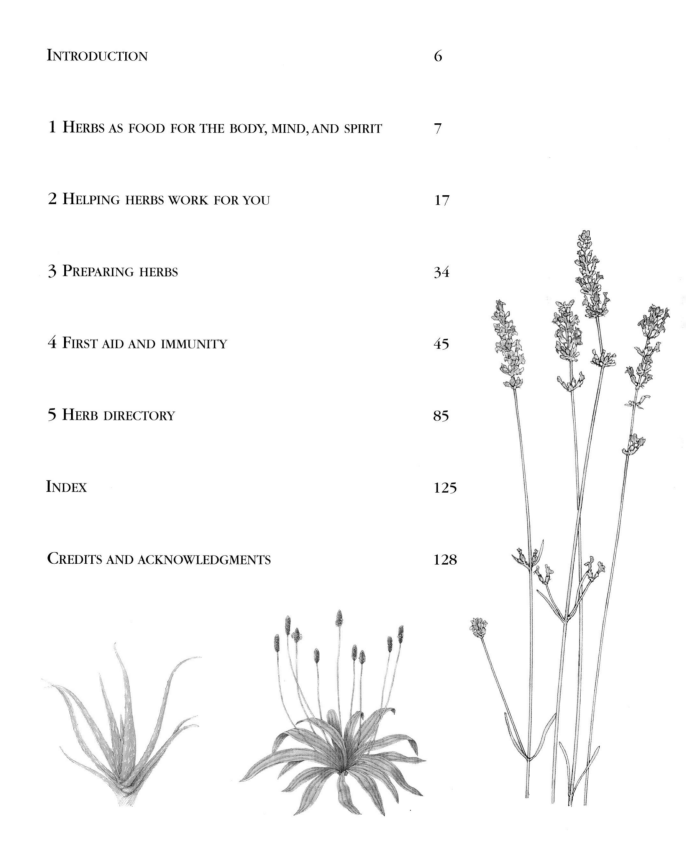

Introduction

Once we would have learned about herbs from our mothers and grandmothers, who would have passed on what they knew from their own experience. They would also have been able to judge how much to teach, according to the ability of the pupil to absorb and make sense of their teaching. Although there are plenty of books about herbs around, they can't give you that, and the complaint of many of my students over the years has been "Books leave you feeling more confused than before: every plant seems to be good for everything."

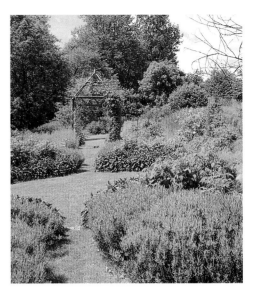

Plants are living things with individual characters.

Well, this is yet another book. The difference between this and many others, however, is that it is a digest rather than an encyclopedia. Instead of trying to cover everything, my aim here is to introduce you to just a few herbs – thirty or so at most – that are at the core of my own practise as a consultant herbalist. Over thirteen years of working with people and plants, I have come to know these herbs intimately, both individually and in combination with others. I know what they can do and would not write a prescription without including at least one. Some are megastars in the world of healing, others are humble garden weeds, but they are all effective.

When you treat someone with a herbal remedy, you are setting up a three-sided relationship: the person who's seeking to improve their health, the herbs that they choose to take and you, introducing the one to the other. You use your knowledge of the patient and the plants to bring them together, and the success of the match depends on how well they get on. Plants are living things, each with their own character, just like us. *Matricaria recutita* (chamomile), for example, may be an unfailing source of comfort to one person, helping them to sleep and calming their worries, while for another it will do nothing at all.

If you want to work with herbs, it is essential that you get to know them, to find out "who" they are and how they behave. Take note of your own reactions to them, too: do you like a particular herb or not? Every practitioner knows that some remedies just don't work for them, while others think that they are heaven-sent. So find out which plants you can work with and be guided by your intuition rather than by what the books say. (And that, of course, applies to this book too!)

All of the remedies I've chosen are ones that you can use with confidence; where there is anything to be cautious about regarding a herb, I shall say so. Some plant remedies can be extremely powerful, and even poisonous, but those are beyond the scope of a self-help book. In any case, to go looking for "magic bullets" is to miss the real treasure that herbal medicine has to offer.

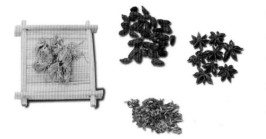

Herbal healers.

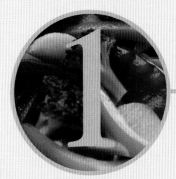

Herbs as food for the body, mind, and spirit

Herbs as food for the body, mind, and spirit

If you drew a line with poisons and drugs (most of which are derived from plants) at one end, and foodstuffs at the other, herbal remedies would come in between, with no dividing lines. At the foodstuffs' end of the scale, there is almost nothing that we eat that does not have some effect on the body beyond that of simply providing nourishment. Take rice, for example: brown rice stimulates the large intestine, promoting good bowel motions, while too much of it can irritate a sensitive or inflamed gut. Any food you can think of will have some effect on you – and you could say, of course, that providing nourishment is a health-promoting function in itself.

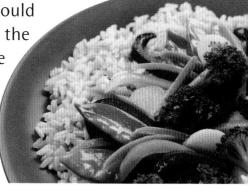

More than just food.

8

At the opposite end of the scale are poisons, some of which can be life-saving in small doses, but, before you reach that extreme you encounter the plants that contain one or more very powerful ingredients, and the drugs that are produced by isolating those ingredients. *Digitalis purpurea* (foxglove) from which the drug digoxin, which is used to treat heart failure, is derived, is a good example. Plants like this are an essential part of herbal medicine, but are best left to the qualified practitioner to prescribe. Besides these, occupying the middle ground are thousands of remedies for you to play with, and these represent the heart of herbal medicine.

Herbs are, on the whole, much more like foodstuffs than drugs. Their action is supportive to the body, lending it strength and feeding it vitality. Many symptoms of illness arise when the body has somehow become unbalanced, often over a long period of time. Humans are generally pretty tough, and we can push our luck a long way before – often suddenly – it decides to desert us. So, when a person gets to the point of deciding to

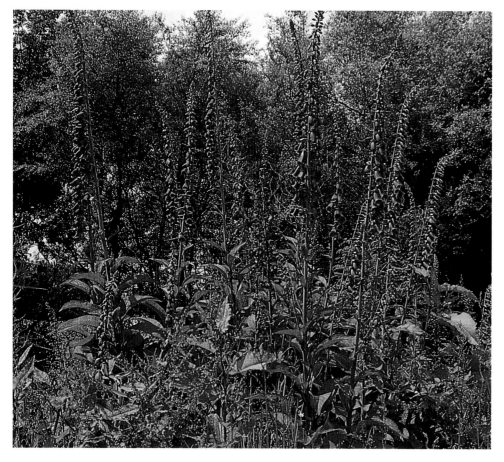

Wild foxglove (*Digitalis purpurea*) aids the heart.

do something about their health problems, nine times out of ten they will already have been living on credit for a while. Their vitality will have been depleted and their reserves will be low. This is when herbs really come into their own.

Do you remember the tonics that doctors used to prescribe? These days, the word "tonic" has become unfashionable in the doctor's office, although "feeling tired all the time" finds its way into patients' case notes more often than ever before. The old-

fashioned tonics often relied heavily on caffeine (so it's probably just as well that they are no longer around), but herbs have far more to offer us than a caffeine buzz or a quick fix for troublesome symptoms. They are tonics in a deeper sense, offering refreshment to body, mind, and spirit, and helping springs that have dried up to flow freely again.

Being tired is an important sign that something is wrong, that something is not being looked after properly. These days, although most of us have plenty

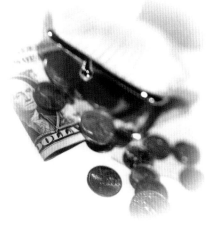

Plenty of this...

... but not enough of this?

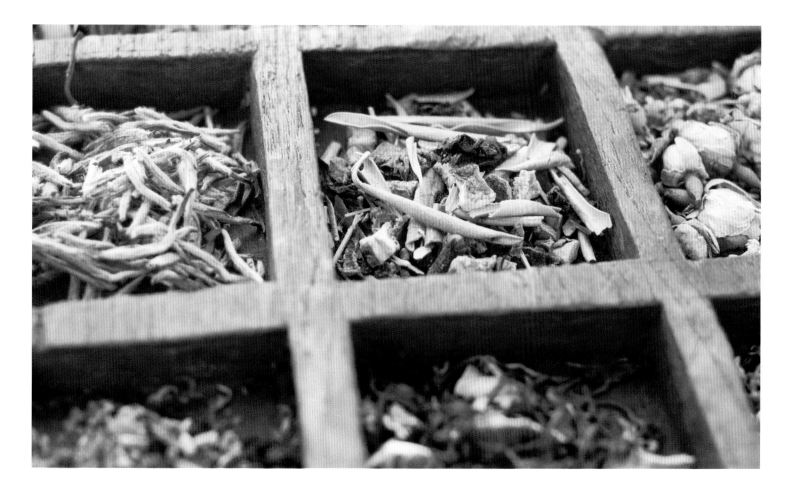

of material goods – food, clothing and other physical comforts – we seem to organize our lives so that we are always running short of other resources that are just as important to our well-being. Some of these are obvious things, like sleep, time and rest. Others are, perhaps, not so obvious, such as the warmth of human contact, a sense of power and purpose in our work, space in which to play and to express ourselves, and constructive ways with which to deal with stress. And the things that we do have plenty of, particularly where food is concerned, may not always be very nourishing: you could say that they feed your face, but not your body.

In many ways, we are behaving like children let loose in a candy store. Until a few thousand years ago, when they discovered agriculture, humans lived mainly on wild plants, supplemented by meat, when they could get it, and the occasional feast of honey or fruit in season. Salt, sweet and high-fat foods were rare and special treats. That's the diet we "grew up" on as humans and, on the whole, it suited us well. Nowadays, however, we're behaving as though we can't get enough treats, as though we need to

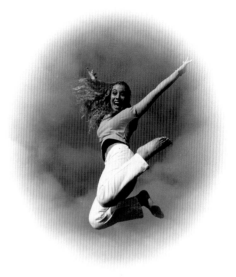

Full of life and on top of the world.

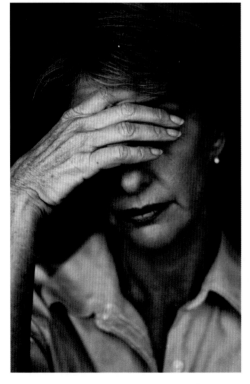

Stress: how do *you* cope with it?

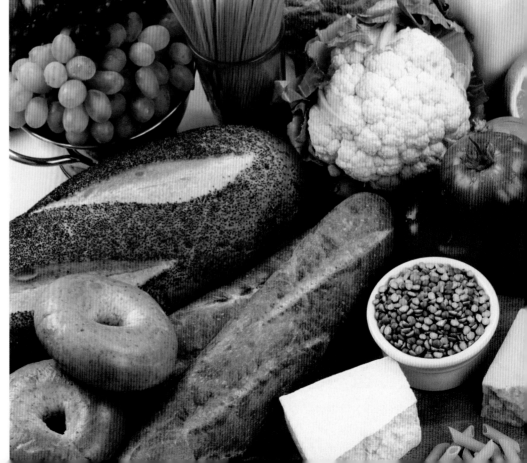

stuff ourselves in preparation for the lean times ahead. And, as you probably know, there's a price to pay for indulging in too many treats at once. In the short-term, you won't feel too well. In the long-term, you'll develop a weight problem and your vital organs – your heart, stomach, pancreas, and liver – will start to feel the strain as your vitality leaks away.

Even the vegetables and fruits that we eat today aren't what they used to be now that we no longer eat much, if any, wild food. Cultivation changes plants, making them yield more, and look better, but causing something to

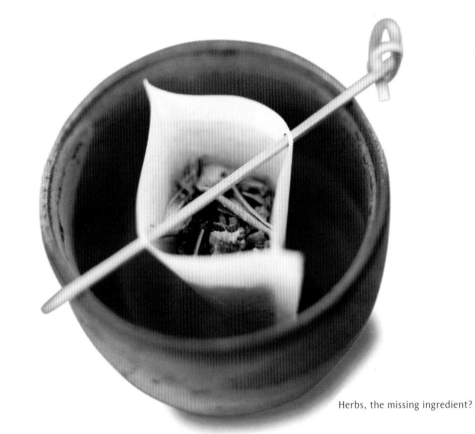

Herbs, the missing ingredient?

be lost in the process. They become blander and less challenging to our taste buds (try chewing a root of wild carrot – *Daucus carota* – and you'll see what I mean). And, as we carefully breed out the bitterness or stringiness, or whatever it is that we don't care for, we are also throwing away some of the ingredients that are more precious than we realize. There are a lot of odd compounds in wild plants – or herbs – that don't seem to play any direct role in nutrition, or, indeed, appear to have any use at all, but the

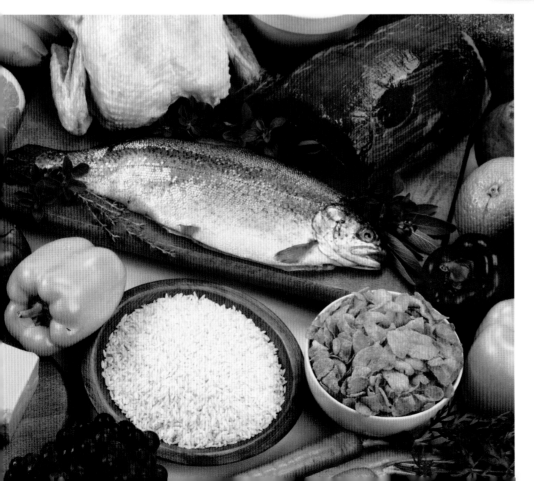

Getting the balance right in our diet.

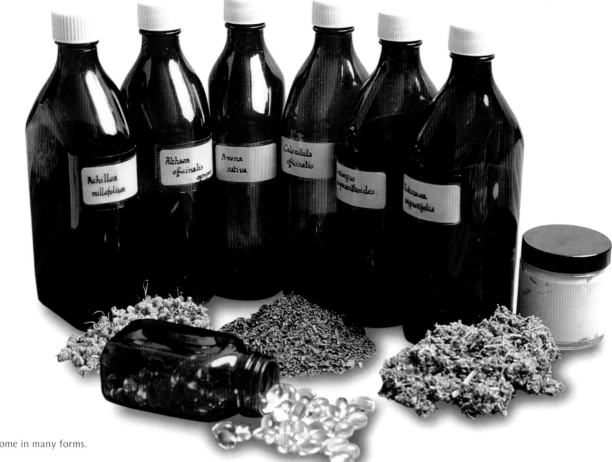

Herbal remedies come in many forms.

evidence is growing that our bodies are missing them. Somehow, in ways that we are gradually coming to understand, they keep our systems awake and alert – in other words, they act as tonic in the true sense of the word. Just as we now know that living in an environment that is too clean and free of germs can lead to our immune systems becoming prone to allergies and intolerances, an overly bland and rich diet can leave your body less than fighting fit.

In other words, we benefit enormously from dietary challenges. The price of too many "comforts" is the sapping of our vital energy. Although we can't go back to being hunter-gath-

erers, we can restore herbs to our diet. The good news is that this doesn't mean having to eat tough and bitter roots, as our ancestors once did. These days you can take herbs as teas, tinctures, or pills – in fact, in almost any way you like. The only problem with taking pills, convenient as they are, however, is that because you can't taste what you are taking, you'll miss out on some of the herbs' beneficial effects (see Chapter 4), and I can guarantee that even if the first taste of some herbal remedies makes you shudder from head to foot, within a week or two your response will have changed dramatically. Stick with the herbs, and you will be rewarded.

NOTE

Let's be clear about one thing: modern medicine does save lives. In places where there is no access to modern drugs and medical techniques, infections are a major cause of death.

Herbal pills, convenient, but not ideal.

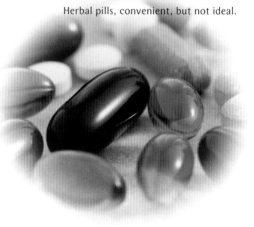

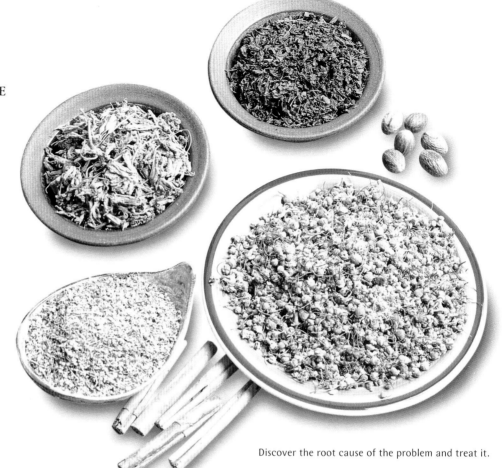

THE PRINCIPLES OF HERBAL MEDICINE

There are some basic principles to be drawn from understanding how herbs work and what they can, and cannot, do. If you take as your starting point these principles, you will not be far off. Your use of herbal medicine will be more effective and economical, and you will develop a real working relationship with plants that goes far beyond simply making use of their healing powers.

1. Herbs are more like food than medicine. Their action tends to be sustaining and supporting. This means that whenever a person has become run down or nutritionally depleted, herbs can be of help. And if you look beyond the immediate symptoms of the illness and try to discover the root cause of the problem, you'll find that depletion will nearly always be a factor. Start by dealing with that, and you will be working at a far deeper level than that of simply trying to get rid of the symptoms.

2. It follows that herbs will be more effective if you look at the factors in the life of the person you are treating that may be leading to illness. In fact, from long experience of working with herbs, I can say with confidence that if they do not do what you expect them to do within, say, three months,

Discover the root cause of the problem and treat it.

something is usually preventing them from doing their job (see chapter 2).

3. Herbal medicine is more about restoring balance than about getting rid of symptoms. For instance, if you have a headache, you might take an aspirin to dull the pain without giving any attention to the cause. That is usually sufficient if it is just a tension headache and you need to get through the day, but what if you keep on getting headaches? In this instance, analyzing what is going on in your body will serve you much better. Maybe there is a source of tension that needs dealing with, maybe you've hurt your neck, maybe you are work-

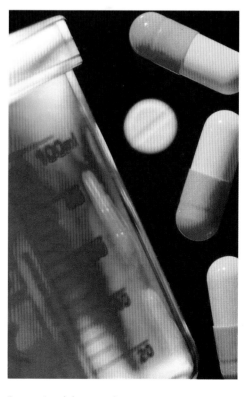

Conventional drugs work on symptoms not causes.

ing under artificial lighting all day, or maybe you're not eating properly . . . Taking aspirin in such circumstances is like sweeping the dirt under the carpet: sooner or later your health will begin to suffer in other ways, too. Herbs, on the other hand, are restorative. Although they're not very effective at killing pain, they're pretty good at tackling whatever is causing it: by boosting your circulation, for example, helping you to cope with stress, or keeping your blood-sugar level constant and so on. Once again, it is very important to remember that this process takes time. Because you didn't get into this state overnight (unless the headaches are the result of an injury), your well-being won't be restored overnight either. Three months is a reasonable period to allow for treating most conditions, and, by the end of that time the problem will either have gone or you should have the sense that your well-being is improving and that things are moving in the right direction. If not, as I warned above, something else will probably need dealing with.

4. The action of herbs is broad rather than specific. Unlike drugs, which generally have a well-defined effect on the body (along with a scatter of side

Dandelion (*Taraxacum officinale)* is a gentle tonic.

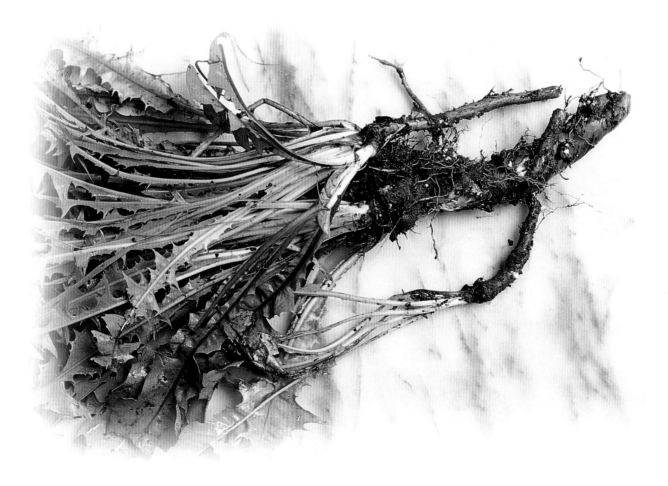

14

Food or medicine? Herbs all support well-being.

you will be able to add to these pictures and sometimes change them. After all, your interaction with these herbs will not be the same as mine.

5. All the above points can be brought together and summed up in one phrase: "whole plants for whole people." Plants, like us, are living things and far too complicated ever to be understood fully. This may be annoying for the scientists among us, but also demands our respect. Although it makes quality control

effects, which are simply the effects that you don't want to occur), herbs tend to work on the individual's constitution rather than the symptoms. This is why, according to so many books about herbs, each plant seems to be good for treating just about everything: you are given a long list of actions, but not much idea of how useful the herb is for treating each of them, meaning that you end up no wiser than before. The solution is to look a little deeper and to try to grasp the essential character of the herb that you are interested in. I have tried to give some indication of the character of each of the herbs in this book and have usually only talked about one or two of the herb's actions, which are the things that I believe it does best. Rather than saying everything that could be said, I have painted my personal picture of each herb, distilled from many years' experience of working with herbs. As you come to know herbs for yourself,

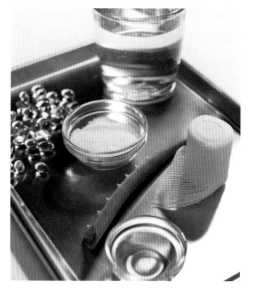

The choice of herbal remedies is endless.

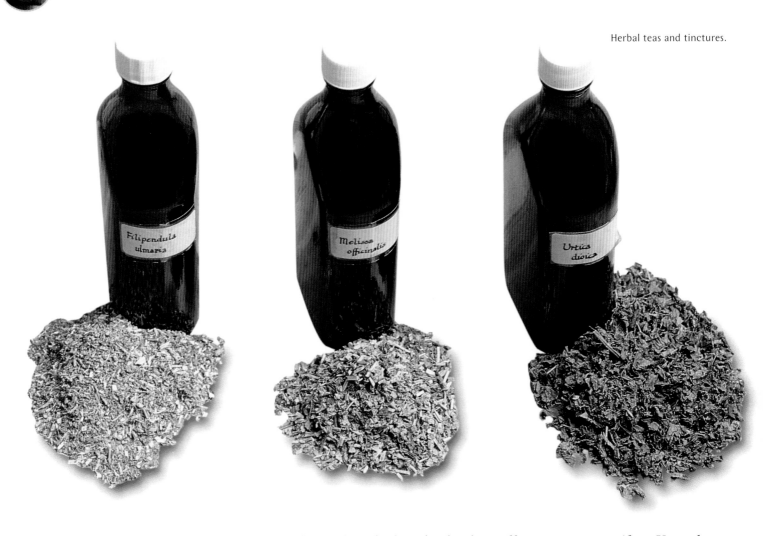

Herbal teas and tinctures.

difficult, and means that you some-times see unexpected reactions between people and plants, this is actually one of the great strengths of herbal medicine. The many constituents of a plant remedy work together, balancing each other, which is one reason why herbal medicine, at least when used within the scope of this book, is so much safer than drug therapy (see *Filipendula ulmaria*, page 95).

6. One last point: when they qualify as professional herbalists, herbal practitioners, like doctors, swear an oath that they will do no harm. If you use the herbs described in this book with proper respect for the cautions and dosages that have been given, you, too, will do no harm, and will certainly do some good. If things are not working out as you feel that they should, if there does not appear to be any significant improvement in the condition that you are treating within a reasonable period of time, or if, for any reason, you feel out of your depth, consult a qualified practitioner.

Don't be afraid to experiment with herbs, however: they have been our faithful allies for longer than any other form of medicine and continue to offer us many gifts. Use them, and enjoy them.

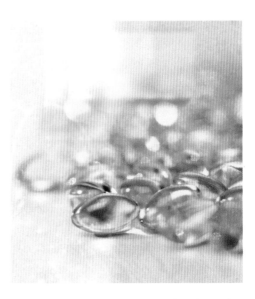

Garlic oil capsules.

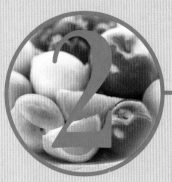

Helping herbs work for you

Helping herbs work for you

The factors that may inhibit the beneficial action of herbs fall into three main categories. The first is diet, or what you put into your system on the physical level. The second is stress, which basically means how you handle what comes your way on other levels. And the third is the sort of disease process that arises from a long-term imbalance, an inherited pre-disposition or an overwhelming trauma that will require either more time to treat or a more aggressive treatment. Let's look at each of these factors in turn.

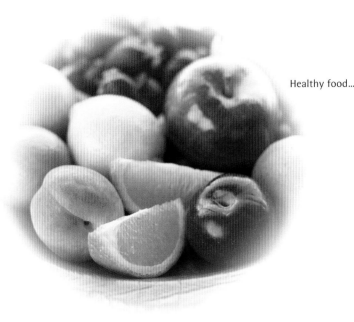

Healthy food...

18

DIET

Although it's not entirely true that you are what you eat, the physical structure of the body does have to be renewed continually. With minor exceptions, the building materials for that renewal process can only gain access to your body by way of your mouth. It makes sense, therefore, to provide your body with the best-quality materials that you can. The bottom line is to choose foods that contain the greatest possible amount of life force, to enable their vitality to feed yours. Vital foods are as fresh and as unprocessed as possible. "Dead" foods, by contrast, will clog up your system and leach away your energy rather than feeding it.

Looking at your diet can sometimes completely turn your idea of what is good for you on its head. Although it may be lower in cholesterol than butter, margarine, for example, is one of

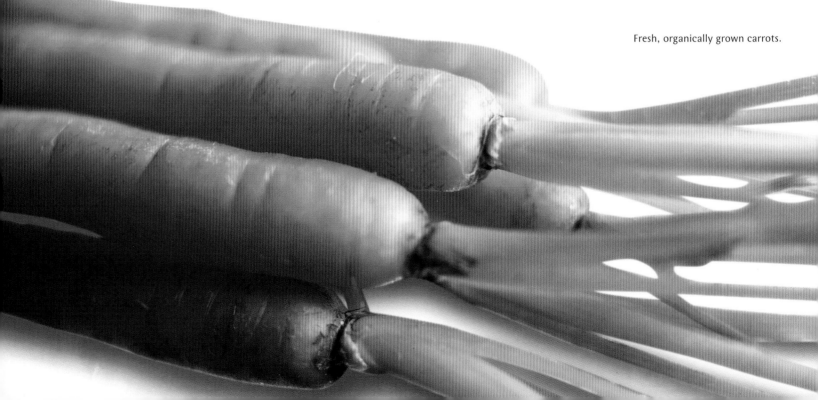

Fresh, organically grown carrots.

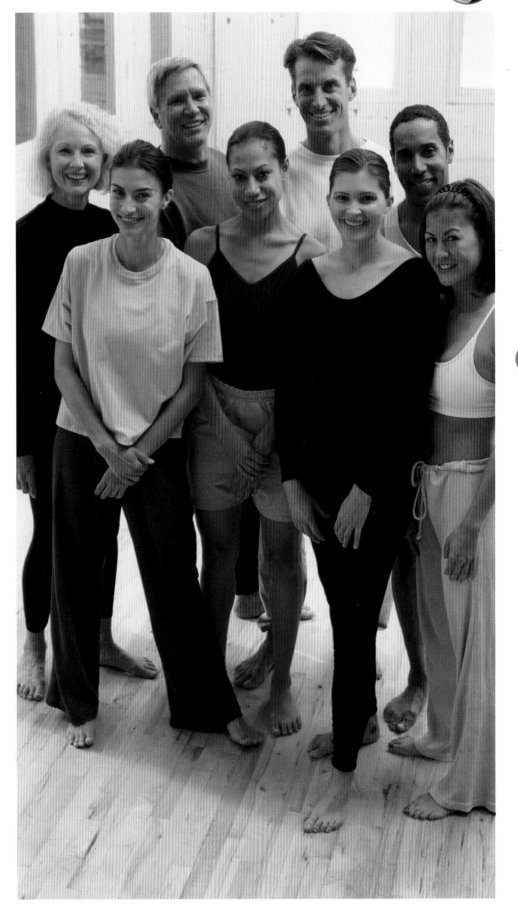

...for healthy people.

the most processed, and "unnatural" foods that we can eat, and it may be healthier to choose butter in some circumstances. Likewise, the organically grown carrots that have stayed in a box for a week at your local whole-food store may contain less life force than their freshly dug, chemically grown counterparts in the supermarket. Don't get me wrong: organic growing methods generally produce foods that are the most supportive of your life force, but storage is important, too, as is preparation.

In general, applying the life-force principle will provide your diet with the kind of base foods that we should all be eating: lots of fresh vegetables and fruit grown without the use of chemical fertilizers or pesticides, and a moderate amount of protein-rich food derived from animals (unless you are vegetarian) that have been non-intensively reared on organically grown foodstuffs. To that base you can add "treats," which are acceptable in moderation, and without which life would be boring.

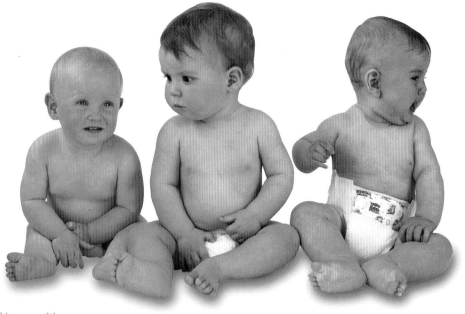

Babies – sensitive

20

A diet like this would keep most people fit and healthy, giving them a long life span, were there no other factors to consider. Food intolerances and sensitivities, and sometimes outright allergies, for instance, are significant problems these days. At least half of my patients have symptoms that can be traced to various foods, the symptoms ranging from obvious digestive troubles like gas or bloating to joint pain and swelling, headaches, and conditions that are hard to pin down, like tiredness, loss of energy, and mental fuzziness.

How do we deal with these problems? On the whole, I do not find allergy-testing very helpful. For every person who has a clear, unvarying response to a particular food – like "I eat beef and twenty minutes later my hands start to swell," as one arthritic patient told me – there are half-a-dozen more who don't. In most cases, people's responses vary from day to day, and from morning to evening, making it hard for them to identify what caused the problem. Allergy-testing will almost certainly yield a long list of foods to be avoided, which, in my experience, usually doesn't result in a big improvement in the person's well-being. Also, keeping to a restricted diet for months at a time can cause its own problems, often disrupting your social life, as well as your nutritional status.

The answer lies at a deeper level. If you have become sensitive to certain foods, ask yourself what this says about the state of your digestion, and about your vitality in general. What is it about your life that has worn you down to the point where you can no longer cope with everyday foods?

Avoiding problem foods in pregnancy can save trouble later.

Note that I am not talking about inherited allergies here. If you were born with an intolerance to eggs or wheat, for example, you will have to think in terms of management rather than cure, although a lot can still be done to strengthen your constitution. But it is uncommon to be allergic to food from birth, although babies may be born with sensitive constitutions. Most of the allergies that manifest themselves early in life begin either with the introduction of certain difficult foods into a child's diet before his or her system is ready to cope with them, or when they are present in the mother's diet while she is pregnant or nursing. In other words, strong reactions to foods, even in babyhood, are an expression of a system that is under stress. And this is something that we can work with.

If you use the kind of supportive, tonic herbs that I have talked about, your digestive system will become stronger and more able to deal with whatever comes its way. It may take a long time – maybe months, or even years – but things will eventually improve. It all depends on how long you have had problems with particular foods, how serious your reactions are, and your willingness to make the necessary changes in your lifestyle, as well as your diet. In the early stages of treatment, it may sometimes be useful to undertake a cleansing fast, but this should always be done under the supervision of a qualified herbal practitioner.

My aim is to get you to the point where you can eat whatever you choose. If you are taking herbs, you will find that your sense of what is good for you and what is not will become sharper. And, because your craving for the foods that will not do your body any favors will become less intense, if you listen to the signals that your body is sending you, you'll be able to heed the warning signs that tell you to avoid them. At the same time, your enjoyment of the food you eat will increase.

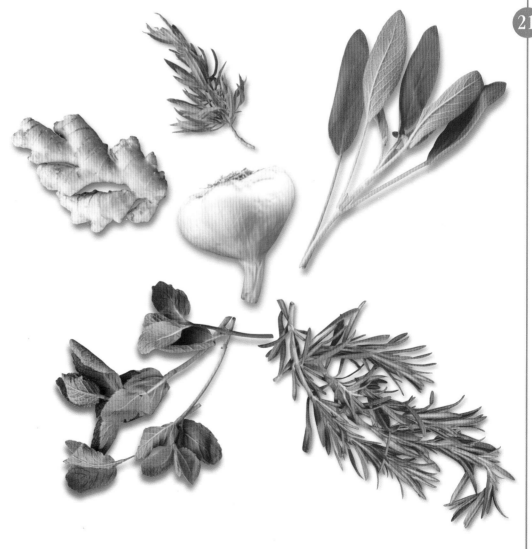

Healthy herbs to support your digestion.

21

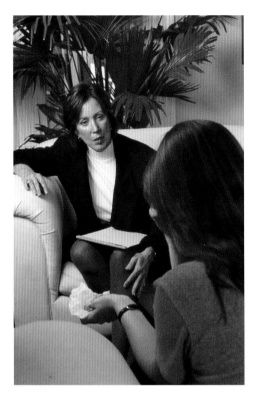

Counseling – learning to deal with stress.

The long-term use of herbs should help you to find and maintain your optimum weight, too, because of the way in which herbs wake up your digestive system and help your body to assimilate nutrients from food. It's important to understand that, if herbs are to be effective, they must be used over the longer term. If you really want to lose weight, taking it slowly and steadily is always best. Although you'll find plenty of herbal slimming mixtures on sale, most of them rely on diuretics and stimulants to achieve a temporary drop in weight, so don't buy them! Instead consult a herbal practitioner to help you set up a weight-loss program that includes dietary changes, herbs and exercise. If you stick with it, you'll get there.

STRESS

Stress is part of being alive and nobody is immune to it. It is how we respond to stress – whether or not we see ourselves as being able to handle it and how much we have to deal with at once – that determines whether we either go with the flow or start to go under.

It is now well understood that a person can go on coping with certain kinds of stress – whether it is eating foods that are difficult to digest or plodding on in a boring job or an unhappy relationship – for a long time. We humans are pretty tough and can endure a lot of damage before the strain starts to show. Then, often suddenly, we stop being able to cope. (This explains why someone who has eaten, say, wheat, with no apparent trouble for the past thirty years can become intolerant to it more or less overnight.) Sometimes you can identify the straw that broke the camel's back, but sometimes it remains a complete mystery. Equally, while a viral infection, for example, a shock, such as an accident or a bereavement, or some other kind of setback, may stand out as an obvious cause of trouble, just as often there may be no clear precipitating cause –

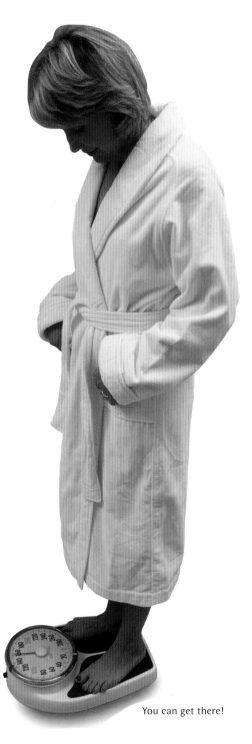

You can get there!

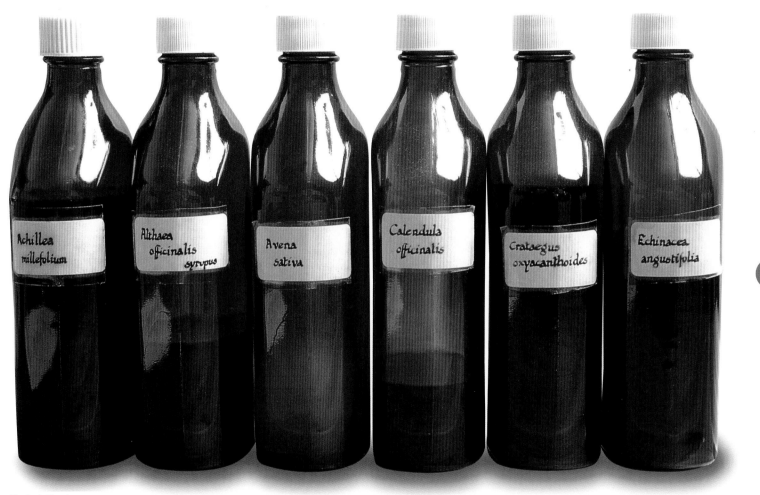

Herbal tinctures.

sometimes the system simply becomes too tired to cope.

When treating someone, it helps to try to identify any sources of stress, even if the person does not intend to do anything about them. There are some things that we are called upon to do in life that are hard to cope with, where the burden is heavy and the rewards small. Many stresses, therefore, need management rather than elimination: caring for an elderly parent or a demanding child, for instance. We know that stress lowers our resistance to illness and our ability to respond flexibly and creatively to challenges. And we also know that while some people seem to thrive on stress and feel more alive under pressure, others find it hard to tolerate. Nevertheless, we all have different breaking points, and if someone has reached the point of experimenting with herbs to try to deal with whatever symptoms have arisen, it is likely that they have heard the warning bells.

Herbs can help you to cope with stress: with their restorative, nourishing qualities, they will make you stronger and feed your fire. They can help you to rise to challenges better, enabling you to hold your own in a demanding work situation, for example, or to keep your temper with your difficult children instead of

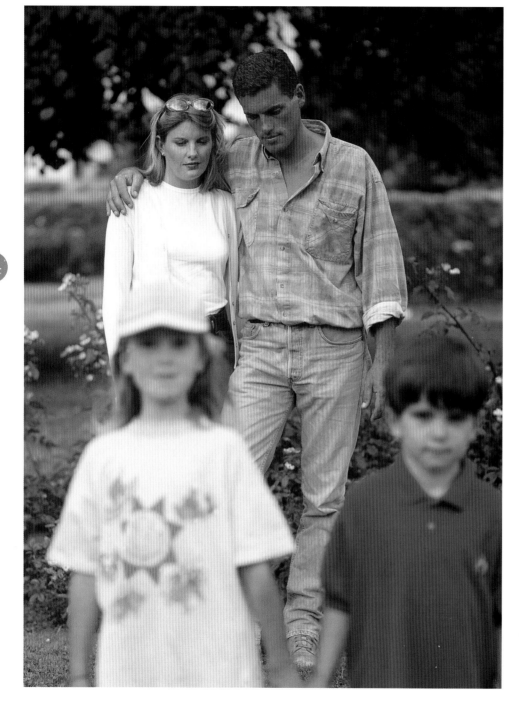

Parenting can be a stressful job at times.

troubles, so that although you can't feel your misery, it remains beneath the surface. Although such drugs can sometimes give you some respite, allowing you to carry on functioning, sometimes they turn people into sleepwalkers. And coming off them is nearly always a slow and difficult business. This is a process that herbs can also alleviate, although it would be a mistake to think of, for example, *Hypericum perforatum* (St. John's Wort) as a herbal subsitute for Prozac, because herbs support your nervous system, enlivening you, rather than putting you to sleep. If you're trying to come off anti-depressants or any other drugs, it's best to have a herbal support system already in place, ideally with the help of a qualified practitioner of herbal medicine, who will change your prescription as you progress (and it can be a rough ride).

Finally, because herbs feed your fire, they can make it harder for you to remain in a situation that is harming you. Sometimes it may be appropriate to hang on in there and keep coping, but, at other times getting out is the right thing to do. When you've been ground down, ending an abusive relationship, leaving a soul-destroying job, dealing with bullies or simply standing up for yourself can be too

losing it. Herbs can encourage you to feel happier and more serene, but not in the way that tranquilizers and anti-depressants work. Taking Prozac or Valium is essentially like throwing a big, thick, soft blanket over your

much to ask. But, of course, not taking this step will cause your self-esteem to drop even further and you'll sink deeper into depression. Conversely, as your brain becomes sharper and you feel more alive, it will become harder to put up with injustices and easier to fight back. To put it another way: if your spirit is strong, not only can you see more choices open to you, but you

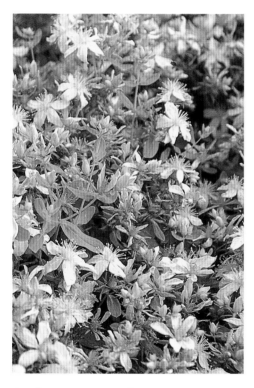

St. John's Wort supports the nervous system.

have more of a sense of your own power to make those choices and carry them through.

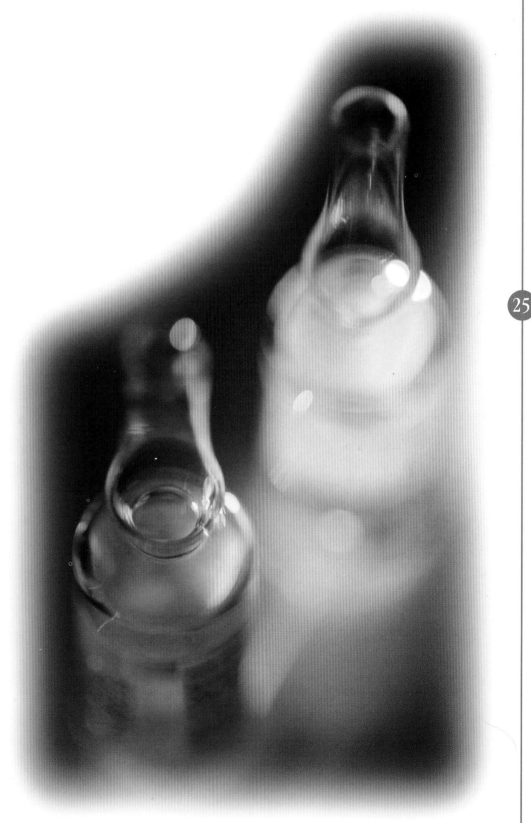

DISEASE

You can't cure everything: although it may take decades to become apparent, people may be born with physical problems. There are also disease processes that cannot be stopped or that lead to irreversible damage within the body. Modern medicine is pushing back the frontiers of disease all the time, but there will always be illnesses, injuries and, of course, death. Wisdom lies in knowing what you can, and cannot, treat, as well as just how much you can do.

Illness is a fact of life.

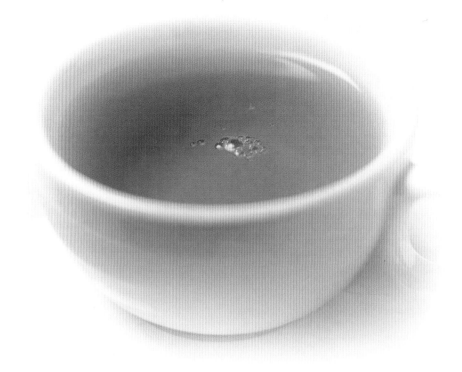

Whatever your condition, there is nearly always something herbs can do.

Having said that, there is nearly always something that herbs can do: because they support your life force, they can help you to bear ill health, even if they cannot always cure it. It is well known that people feel more

26

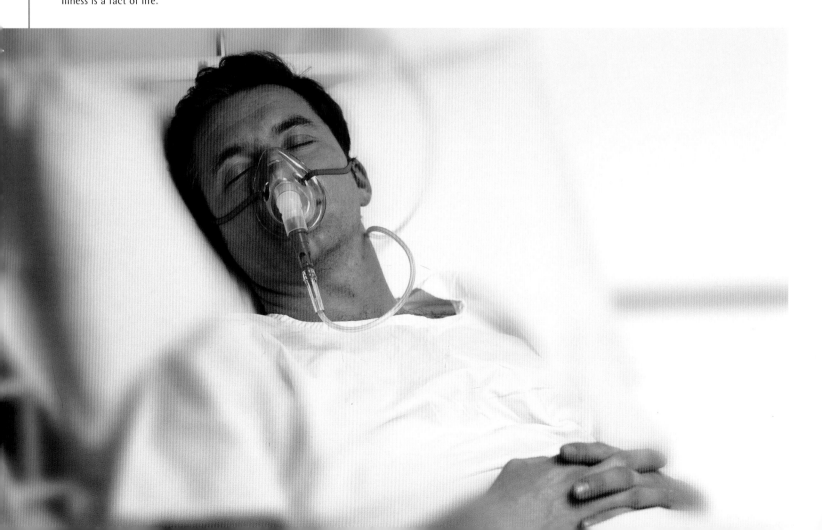

pain when they are tired, run down or depressed, which means that working on these problems can greatly improve their general condition. Because herbs don't work in a suppressive way, they are not so good at providing strong pain relief, although they can have a beneficial effect on whatever it is that has given rise to the pain. Inflammation, for example, can respond well to herbal medicine.

If you look deeper, beyond the obvious symptoms, you will find a role for herbs to play when someone is suffering from a disease. One very valuable job that they can perform, for example, is supporting the patient when he or she is taking conventional drugs or undergoing surgery. Herbs are tonic for the liver, too, helping it to cope with the burden of chemotherapy. They stimulate circulation, thus speeding up tissue-healing. They improve digestion, which often suffers from the side effects of drugs, and help to keep the body well nourished. Herbs also improve the patient's ability to cope with the stress and anxiety of everything.

If you are combining taking herbs with conventional drugs, it is always best to let your doctor know what you are taking: apart from any beneficial effects, there may be interactions or

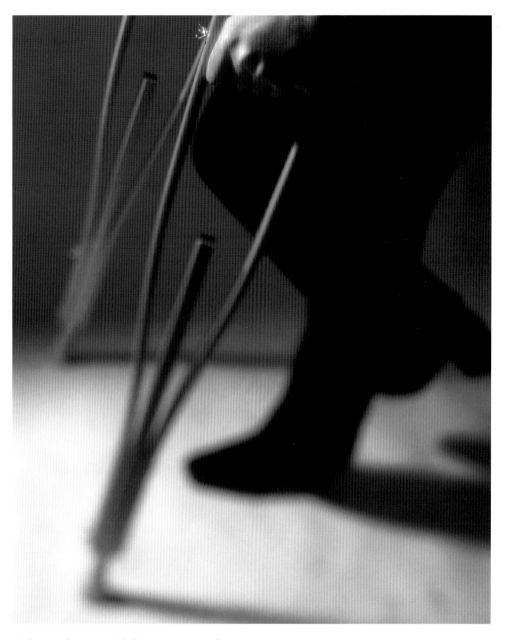

Herbs can play a part in helping you recover from an injury.

overlaps that you don't want. If you are diabetic and dependent on insulin, for example, taking herbs that lower your blood-sugar level could destabilize your condition. In addition, some herbs, notably *Hypericum perforatum* (St. John's Wort), speed up the rate at which the body metabolizes some drugs, making them less effective. So, if a drug regime is involved, this is an area best left to a qualified herbalist, who will know

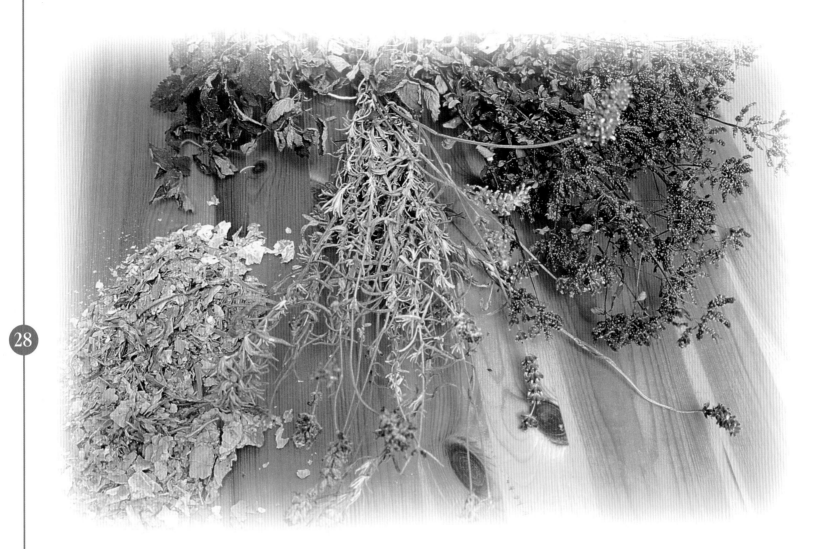

Dried herbs for making teas and tisanes.

how to work around it and when to leave well alone.

Likewise, if you're not sure about anything, or you've been using herbs and haven't had the response that you were hoping for, consult either a herbalist or a doctor because it may be that you haven't recognized a problem or it may be that more aggressive or intensive treatment is needed. Resorting to orthodox methods like drugs and surgery – which can, and do, save lives – doesn't mean that you've failed as a herbalist. Instead of attacking each other's weaknesses, practitioners of all branches of the healing arts are slowly learning to work together and celebrate each other's strengths.

And it is my belief that the healing arts will truly come of age in the coming decades as modern discoveries take their place alongside the older therapies.

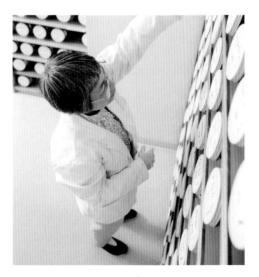

When combining remedies consult a professional.

"GREEN" MEDICINE

Is herbal medicine "green" medicine? Well, yes, up to a point. One of the reasons that people often give for choosing herbal medicine is that it is "natural." And because "natural" is frequently interpreted as meaning wholesome, in harmony with the Earth and not meddled with by humans, it follows that it must be good for us. There is some truth in this, of course, otherwise this book would not be worth writing, but it's not the whole truth.

The first, and most obvious, thing to remember is that not everything that nature produces is good for us. There are plenty of highly effective poisons in the plant world, and plenty more which, although they may not kill you outright, would certainly not enhance your life force. We therefore need to approach plants with respect and reverence and remember that they are not there entirely for our benefit.

My second point is that we are not using herbs in anything like their natural state, that is, unless we are

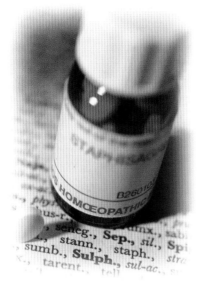

Homeopathic pills.

picking their leaves directly off living plants. Even drying herbs removes more than just water. It's a compromise that we have to make when we want to use herbs that are out of season, that originate from a distant land, or that are not easy to digest in their natural state. That apart, many of the preparations that you can buy have had all sorts of things done to them – extraction using heat or chemicals, the discarding of unwanted parts and the addition of preservatives, flavors or colors, for instance – many of which don't enhance the healing potency of the natural plants.

Commercial preparations are likely to be more highly processed and packaged than those supplied by a herbal practitioner, because such sophisticated handling adds value –

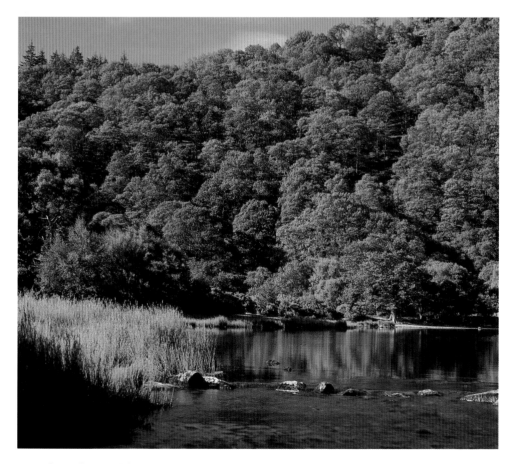

Natural remedies: good for nature or good for us?

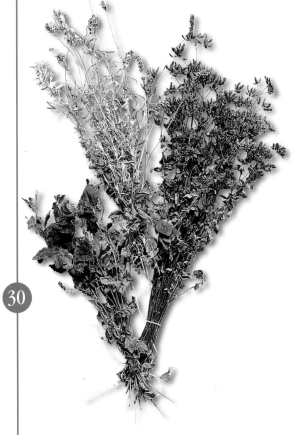

Gathered from the wild...

...or grown to be used?

30

not to you, the consumer, but to the producer. If you really want a "natural" medicine, the golden rule is to use preparations that are as simple as possible. To ensure this, grow or gather what you can and make your own remedies. Alternatively, buy organically grown herbs and choose dried herbs or tinctures rather than pills and expensive, over-the-counter products. In addition, most herbalists will be happy to supply you with teas to drink for pleasure, as well as for healing, once you are on their patient list.

And so to my third point. In the course of their hunting and gathering, our early ancestors used whatever came their way – animal, vegetable or mineral – for healing. Ingredients were chosen for a variety of reasons, some entirely logical and carefully worked out, others purely magical and still others for reasons that fell somewhere in between the two. By means of a process that is probably deeply rooted in the human psyche, our ancestors often came to believe that certain medicines that were rare or difficult to find had more value than those that were common and readily available. Well, not much has changed since then. Although we now grow a lot of herbs for medicinal and other uses, we continue to believe

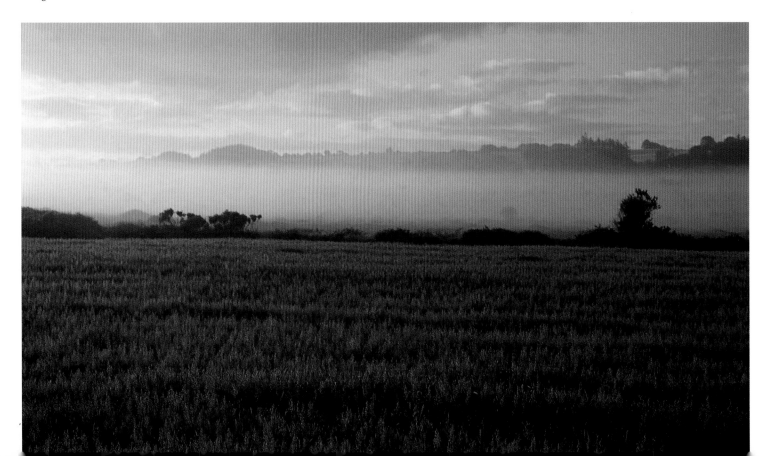

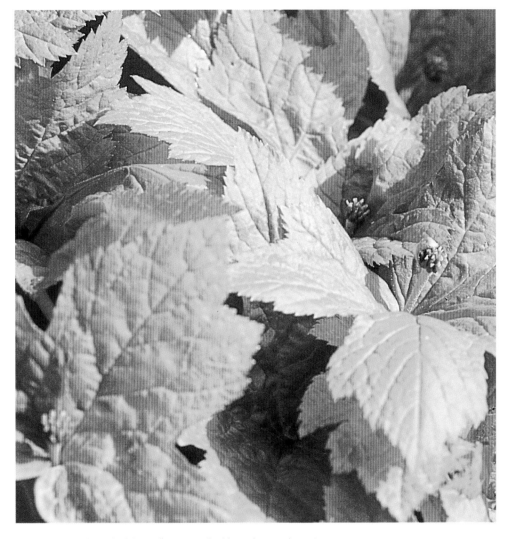

Hydrastis canadensis (goldenseal) is now a highly endangered species.

ist I know uses it now, but many do still work with *Hydrastis canadensis*, goldenseal, which is also extremely rare.) Yet there are alternatives: nature is infinitely generous and there is no need to fall into the trap of believing that only one particular plant can do the trick. You can get stuck in this kind of belief through having successfully used a herb once or having been taught about its qualities by someone whom you respect.

Because the bottom line is not to give you information, but to sell you a product, the most dangerous type of mental imprinting comes from advertising. Remember that it is in the advertiser's interest to talk up the powers of a herbal product, to use the lure of the exotic and to play on your anxieties about illness. I recently had a visit from a patient who had been seeing me for some time for stress-related problems. She arrived full of excitement, carrying a handful of print-outs from the Internet about a herb that appeared to offer the solution to all of her troubles. The herb was *Hypericum perforatum* (St. John's Wort). When I told her I had been including it in her prescription from the start of her treatments with me, she was disappointed, as though the herb itself had somehow let her

that wild plants have greater healing virtues than cultivated ones. We are easily seduced by the exotic, the rare and the special, and we undervalue what grows in our own yards.

Most people are aware of the damage that has been done to some wildlife species – tigers, rhinos and seahorses are probably among the best known – by the human search for

medicines that either don't work at all or don't do anything that couldn't be done by less precious and fragile ingredients. Plants, however, don't make the headlines in the same way. If *Cypripedium pubescens* (Lady's slipper orchid) has been gathered almost to extinction because it makes a good treatment for insomnia and anxiety, who really cares? (Actually, no herbal-

Ready to drink.

nothing but the whole herb will do, and wild plants are regarded as being more potent than "tame" ones. And it's gold-rush time for the "nutraceutical" industry. Demand is booming, and every time that the spotlight falls on a potentially new herbal superstar – preferably one used in the shamanic traditions of some colorful tribe in an exotic location – a process begins that threatens to kill off both the plant itself and the traditions within which it is used. To start with, supplies are bought from people who have been

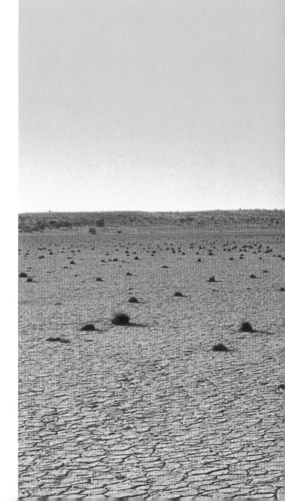

down. My advice is, therefore, to be wary about what you read in advertisements or on the Internet: the dream factory is constantly churning out new material, but real information is not so easy to come by.

The cost of herbal medicine – to the planet, as well as to those of us who use it – is rising. This is partly because increasing numbers of people are turning to herbs, either as an alternative to orthodox drugs, or for use in combination with them. The so-called "nutraceutical" industry (which produces herbal and dietary supplements), which is growing at a phenomenal rate, is, ironically, having a far more destructive impact on the environment than the manufacturers of pharmaceutical drugs. Although about 80 per cent of drugs are derived from plants, the companies that produce them make every effort either to synthesize the vital ingredients, or to obtain their raw materials from growers who deliver them reliably. For many producers of herbal medicines, on the other hand, gathering the herb for local use, who know when, and which parts to harvest and where the best plants grow, and who will leave sufficient plants to enable more to grow next year. Demand soon outstrips that source, however, and as the price of the herb increases, more and more people go out hunting for this treasure. As a result, whole colonies are plundered, habitats are destroyed, and all sorts of other plants are mixed in with the superstar herb to boost the yield. Ultimately, the herb thus becomes unavailable to the very people who have used it for centuries, while, in affluent countries, consumers pay a high price for a glossily packaged product.

Although some herbs have been lost to us and some local economies have been de-stabilized beyond recovery, this is not just a story of gloom and disaster. In the best cases, companies with a

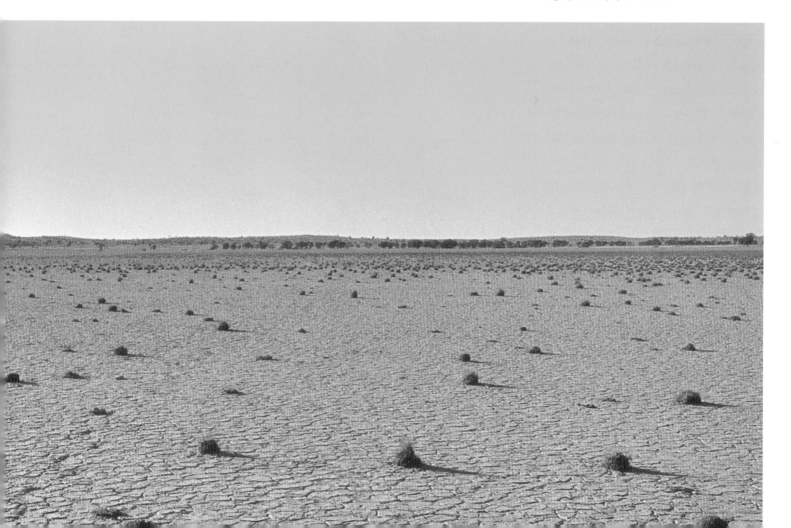

Surfing the net: it's a jungle out there...

A high price to pay for health?

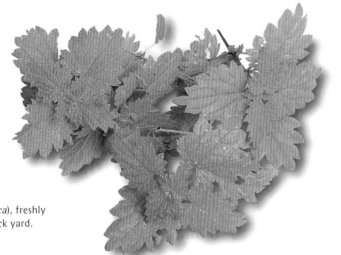

Nettles (*Urtica dioica*), freshly picked from the back yard.

social conscience work together with local people to grow and harvest herbs in a sustainable way. After all, this serves everybody's needs: the company receives a regular supply of herbs that is reliable both in terms of quantity and quality, while the growers are nurturing a valuable source of income. Things may not be the same as they once were, but if we want access to the traditional medicines of other cultures, it is a change that we have to accept.

So where does this leave us, the consumers? In our search for "green" medicine, we have to learn that we cannot simply grab what attracts us, like children let loose in a toy store. Instead, we have to grow up a little. For me, if healing is bought at a cost to a community on the other side of the world, and at cost to the planet, then

the price is too high. We need to recognize that there may be weeds growing all around us, such as *Urtica dioica* (nettle) or *Taraxacum officinale* (dandelion) in Europe and America, that have just as much to

offer us as some of the more glamorous and highly publicized herbs from elsewhere in the world.

And when we do choose to use such herbs, we must do so with an awareness of our responsibilities. This means buying from companies that are committed to sustainable methods of production, accepting that we can only afford to use wild plants if they are common and not jumping on the latest bandwagon without giving any thought to the cost involved.

The world is much too small a place for that.

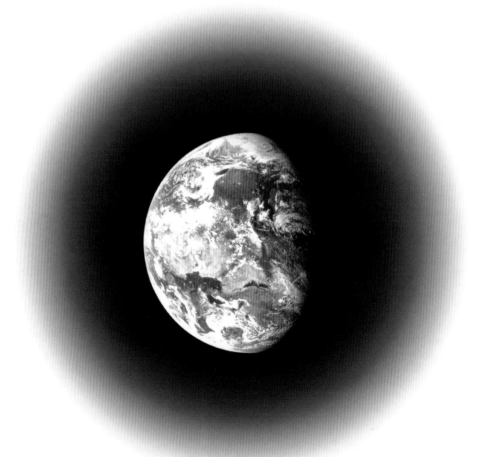

Keeping the planet green.

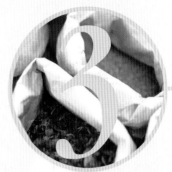

Preparing Herbs

Preparing herbs

The best way of starting to get to know wild plants is to go out exploring with someone with experience. There's no better, or more satisfying, way to learn about them than to spend some time with someone who knows – and loves – plants. So, if you are lucky enough to know a herbalist or plant enthusiast, tag along. If you don't, look out for advertisements for "herb walks" or classes on herbal medicine. Books and other teaching aids are also essential, of course, but there's no substitute for the handing down of knowledge from person to person. That's the way it's always been.

Dried herbs, ready for use.

That said, you must acquire a good guide book for plant identification, and learn to recognize them with confidence before trying out any plants - either on yourself or anybody else. A lot of plants will do nothing for your health, while some are definitely harmful (our early ancestors learned this by trial and error a long time ago, so we shouldn't need to go over that ground again). You'll soon discover that plants of the same species can look very different depending on where they are growing, the time of year, their state of health and so on, but you will also develop the ability to recognize them under any conditions. Just like animals, most plants are pretty distinctive once you've developed an eye for their characteristics.

When it comes to gathering herbs to use as remedies, the key is to choose plants that are as healthy-looking as possible. You are hoping that they will share their vitality with you, so don't pick specimens that look as though they are in trouble or are growing too near a road or another source of pollution. And when you do find what you want, don't be greedy: leave enough to enable the colony to continue to thrive so that there will still be a supply for you next year.

A herb garden is an attractive, as well as useful, addition to any yard.

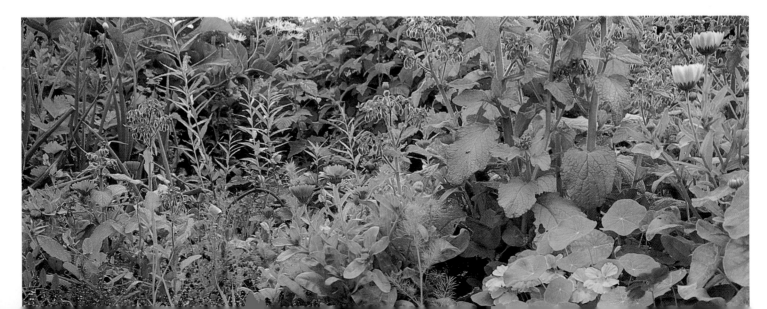

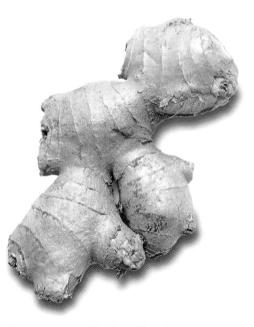

Fresh ginger root (*Zingiber officinalis*).

WHEN TO GATHER HERBS

There are many factors to consider regarding when best to gather herbs: the time of year, the phases of the moon, the time of day, and weather conditions.

The time of year

Plants that grow in temperate zones tend to grow fast in spring, to flower in summer, to set fruit or seed in autumn and to die back, or at least to slow down in growth, in winter. If you want to gather leaves and stems, you'll accordingly find them at their peak in spring and early summer, before the flowers appear. Picking off buds before they can flower will prolong your harvest of leaves: if you're a fan of nettle (*Urtica dioica*) soup, for example, a little judicious pruning of your nettle crop should keep you in tender young greens for the most part of the year.

Flowers are best picked just as they begin to open. Seeds should be dry, ripe and ready to fall. Late autumn and winter, when the vitality of the plant has sunk beneath the earth, are the best times for digging up roots.

Seeds of change...

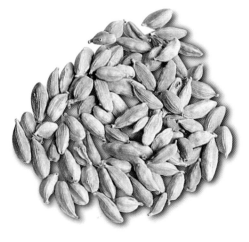

Cardamom

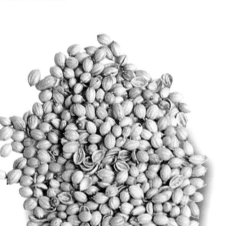

Coriander

Celery

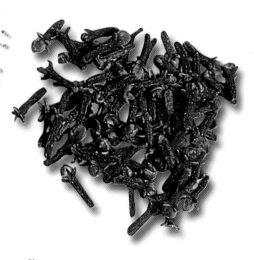

Cloves

Caraway

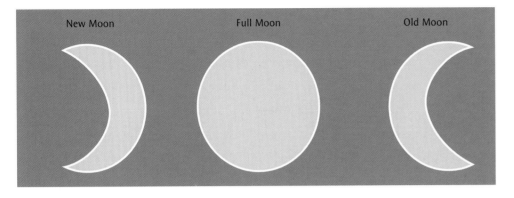

New Moon   Full Moon   Old Moon

The time of day

The chemical constituents of a plant change subtly from hour to hour (a fact that plagues the quality controllers of the herb-processing industry, but inspires reverence in the respectful herbalist). Briefly, the aerial parts are at their best in the morning, after the dew has dried and before the sun has burnt off too much moisture. Roots come into their own in the evening and at night.

Weather conditions

Try not to gather leaves and flowers when they are wet because they will both be hard to dry and likely to develop mould. Remember, too, that gathering them in intense sunlight will decrease the amount of precious volatile oils within your sample.

The phases of the moon

Like all other living things, plants consist largely of water, which means that they respond to the pull of the moon. Seeds germinate better if you sow them a few days before the moon is full. It's not easy to quantify, but the potency of the aerial parts of a plant – the leaves, stems, flowers and seeds – is likely to be greater when the moon is waxing, whereas the root will be at its best when there is a new moon. These considerations are less important for medicinal than for magical purposes, but then the dividing line between the two has always been hazy.

FOOTNOTE

Despite having given all of that advice, I recognize that you are most likely to go gathering when you have the time and when it isn't raining. Aim to gather herbs in ideal conditions, but don't become too hung up on it. Having the will to gather herbs is more important than getting it exactly right.

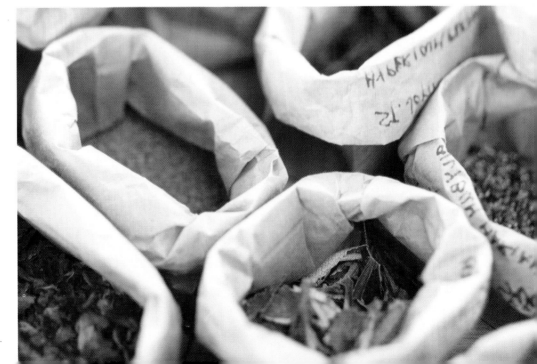

Dried herbs keep best in bags.

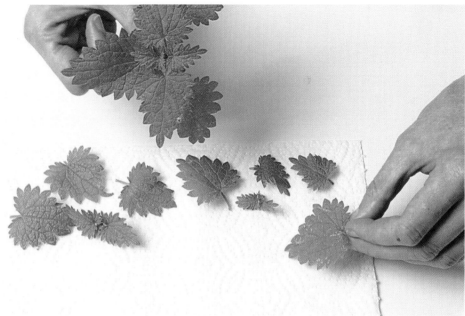

Laying out nettle leaves for drying.

DRYING AND STORING HERBS

Most herbal preparations require dried herbs. Once dried, the majority of herbs will keep for at least a year, which means that they will be available whenever you want to make them into teas, tinctures, creams, syrups or anything else. Recipes tend to assume that you are using dried herbs, so if you are using fresh ones, you'll have to allow for the extra water (about four times as much) that they contain.

Herbs must be dried as quickly as possible in order to preserve their medicinal qualities. Too much heat will parch them and dry up their volatile oils, while exposing them to too much light is also not good. In most households, the ideal place to dry herbs is on slatted shelves in a warm, dry cabinet, with the herbs laid out on sheets of paper and the door left open so that the air can circulate.

Remember to cut up any roots and woody stems before you dry them because this will be difficult to do once they've dried.

Cutting up dandelion roots.

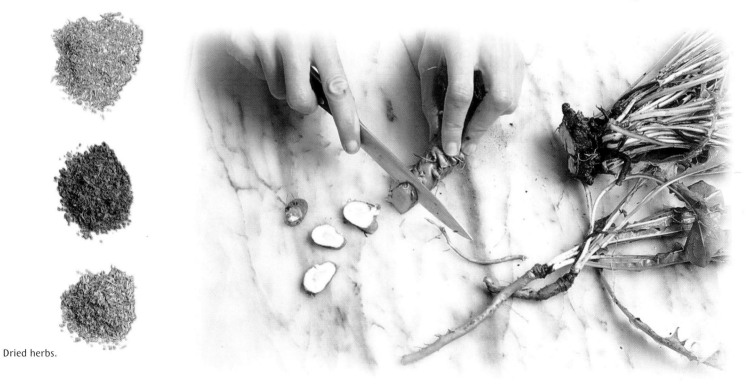

Dried herbs.

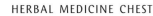

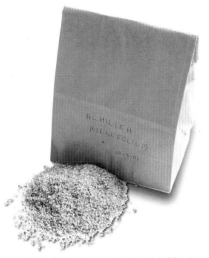

Paper bags, the best way to store dried herbs.

and will crumble at your touch, but their colors should be bright and their scent, if any, fresh and strong. But where should you store them? Again, the prettiest option is the worst: herbs that are sealed in clear glass jars and kept near the stove or on a windowsill will soon become useless for anything except feeding the compost pile. They may have been dried, but they still contain water, and, if they are kept in a sealed container, condensation will develop, and they will become moldy. Dried herbs are best kept in brown paper bags - clearly labeled with the name of the herb, the part collected, and the date - and stored somewhere cool, out of direct sunlight.

Probably the worst thing that you could do is to hang up your herbs in decorative bunches above the stove, where they'll attract grease, dust and insects, bits will drop off them and they'll be at the mercy of the sunlight and heat. They may convince your neighbors that you're a healer, but they won't do much for you.

Drying should be completed within two to three days. If they have dried well, leaves and flowers will be crisp

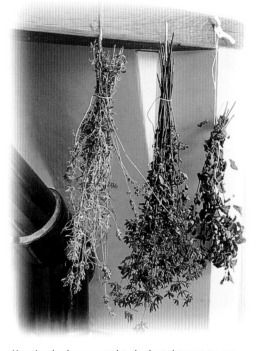

Hanging herbs are good to look at, but not to use.

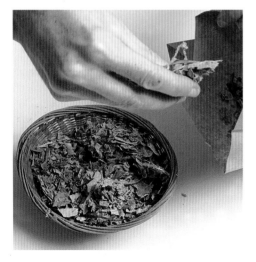

Crumbling the leaves after drying.

Clear glass jars may be pretty, but they're not very practical.

Herbal preparations

The list of herbal preparations is endless, and is limited only by your own inventiveness. Through the ages, people used whatever came to hand as a means of introducing herbs to patients' bodies and must quickly have discovered that it is usually easier, more effective, and more palatable to prepare a remedy rather than asking someone to eat fresh herbs. A few plants, such as *Tanacetum parthenium* (feverfew) are best taken fresh, but most will happily lend their healing qualities to whatever carrier you choose.

For simplicity's sake, I shall explain three basic ways of preparing herbs – as teas or tisanes, tinctures and creams – all of which can be adapted to suit your needs.

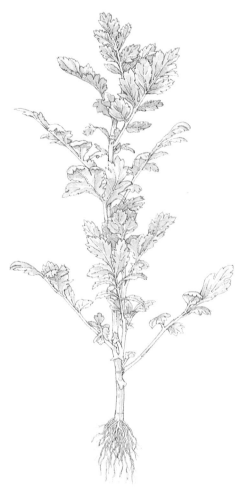

To treat migraines, *Tanacetum parthenium* (feverfew) is best used fresh.

Teas or tisanes

A herbal tea is simply an extract of herb steeped in water, usually hot. For leaves and flowers, it is enough to pour boiling water over them and then leave the tea to brew for about five minutes (this is called an infusion). For tough stems and roots, stronger measures are needed: they must be placed in water and boiled for about fifteen minutes to make a decoction (or "soup" in the Chinese system). Either way, you need about 1oz/30g of dried herb (or 4oz/120g of fresh herb) to half a liter of water to make a standard medicinal extract.

Because dosage is not that critical for any of the herbs that I shall be discussing, don't worry about exact measurements, except where mentioned for a specific herb. This means that you can experiment with the strength of your tea to make it more (or less) palatable, according to your

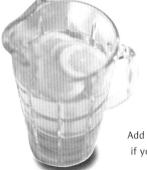

Add lemon, if you like.

taste. You can also mix herbs together, add some lemon or a pinch of cinnamon or ginger or even disguise the taste with fruit juice. Aim to drink two to three cups of herb tea a day.

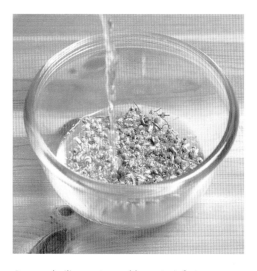

Pour on boiling water and leave to infuse.

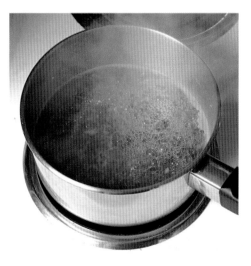

Boiling roots or stems.

Tinctures

A modern invention, tinctures are usually made with herbs and a mixture of water and alcohol or glycerol. Alcohol is usually the herbalist's favorite because it is an excellent extractor of the active ingredients of most plants, while its strength means

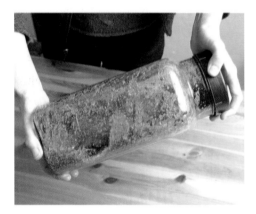

Shaken, not stirred – herbs, vodka and water.

that your dose of herbal medicine will come in a teaspoon rather than a cup (good news in the case of some of the stronger-tasting herbs).

Tinctures can be kept for a year or more, unlike teas, which must be used within twenty-four hours. Although they are obviously not suitable for recovering alcoholics, or for anyone who has a sensitivity or an aversion to alcohol, they perform well for most

people. The simplest way to make a tincture is first to start with a liter of good-quality vodka (the proportion of alcohol to water in vodka is just about right for extracting the active principles of most herbs). Pour the vodka into a large glass jar with a lid, add about 4oz/120g of dried herb – the water content of fresh herb would upset the alcohol/water balance – and shake up the ingredients. Then replace the lid and leave the jar to stand (out of direct sunlight) for two weeks, shaking or turning it daily. At the end of that time, strain off the tincture into dark-colored glass bottles and label them with the date and name of the herb or herbs that they contain.

The standard adult dosage is three 5ml teaspoons of tincture daily, usually taken on an empty stomach. For people over seventy or under seven, halve the dosage; for babies, a few drops can be enough. Again, it is hard to be precise: some people seem to

Taking the medicine.

need bucketfuls before the tincture has any effect, while others are sensitive to tiny doses. On the whole, the person taking the remedy is the best judge of the quantity required.

All the herbs described in this book may be taken as either teas or tinctures, with a few exceptions which I have dealt with individually. In general, the flowery and leafy herbs are more pleasant as teas, while I would recommend using the less palatable ones as tinctures only. Experiment, and decide for yourself!

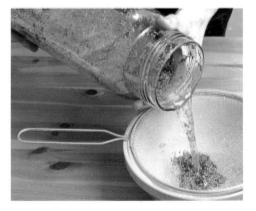

Strain the tincture through a sieve or some muslin.

Creams

You could use a tea or a tincture with which to rub or wash the skin, but a cream base is needed if the preparation is to stay on the skin. What you use as a base depends on what you need the cream to do. If you want it to remain on the skin to act as a barrier – for hands that are exposed to harsh detergents, for instance – or to carry the active ingredients without disappearing too quickly (a chest rub to help an asthmatic patient to breathe more easily, perhaps) then the base must not be soluble in water. It will feel greasy, and will not be capable of being absorbed by the skin. If you want a light cream that will be quickly absorbed, on the other hand, the

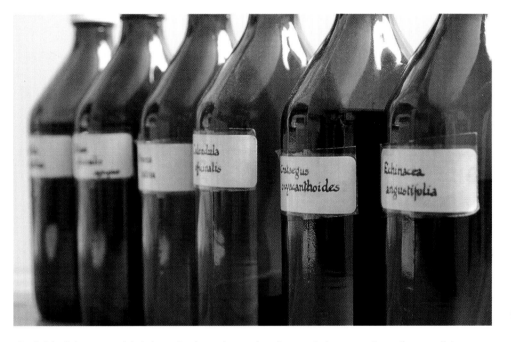

The finished tinctures – label them clearly, and store them in a cool place away from direct sunlight.

base should be largely water-soluble. In practice, a useful base will be a mixture of both types, being fairly solid in the jar, but rapidly dissolving into the skin when applied. Although you could happily experiment with creams forever, there follows a quick run-through of some of the more popular bases.

Until recent times, the mainstay of homemade remedies were animal-based fats, such as lard, butter or goose grease. Although traditional, these do not keep very long and are also unacceptable to vegetarians and vegans. Nowadays, we have a mineral-based alternative in petroleum jelly, and other products also derived from petroleum. These are both "clean" and keep well, but may contain preservatives that can irritate sensitive skin. The natural complement to herbal remedies is the wide range of vegetable oils. Some, such as sunflower

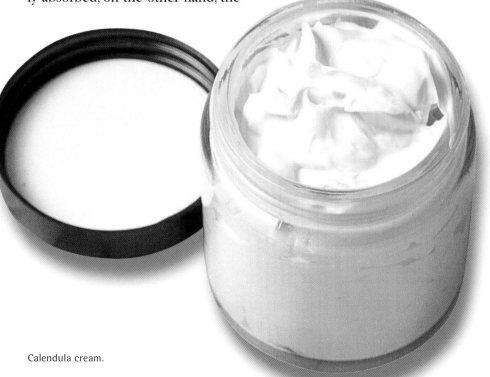

Calendula cream.

and grape seed oil, are simply neutral carriers, while others bring their own qualities to the product. If you want add its own medicinal action. Lavender oil, for example, will enhance the anti-inflammatory action of a cream, while thyme or tea-tree oil will endow it with additional anti-infective properties.

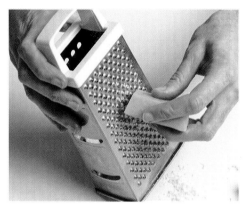
Grating beeswax.

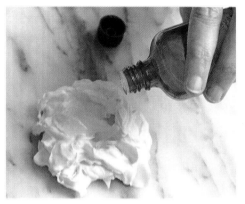
Adding essential oil.

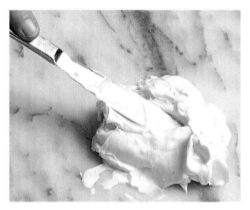
Mixing oil and cream.

44

your cream to be moisturizing, for example, you could use avocado or coconut oil in the base, but if you want it to be anti-inflammatory, evening primrose oil would be an excellent choice.

Whatever oil you choose, it must be combined with something more solid so that you end up with a cream or ointment. The usual choices are beeswax (for non-vegans) or cocoa butter, and the more of each you add, the heavier and longer-lasting your preparation will be. The finishing touch is to add a few drops of an essential oil, which will both help to preserve the final product and

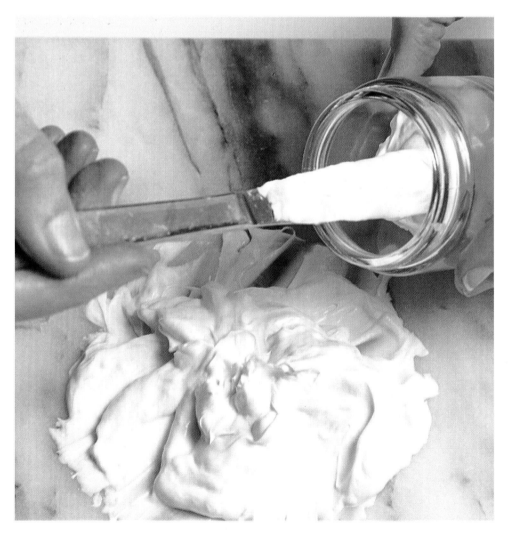
Spooning cream into a jar.

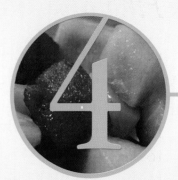

First aid and immunity

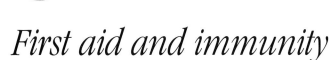

First aid and immunity

Herbs act on two levels. The first, the deeper level, is that of rebalancing and restoring your vitality, the special strength of herbal medicine. As long as you are alive, there is a vital force within you that is always working toward integration, toward wholeness. If that vital force is strong, problems are resolved and healing occurs swiftly; illness, if it comes, will be acute and pass quickly, leaving your system feeling refreshed (see "Feed a fever?", page 64). Herbs are our allies in the task of nurturing our vitality, and replenishing it when it burns low. This task, as we have seen, is a slow and careful business; the "magic bullets" of the pharmaceutical industry don't have much place in herbal medicine.

A cry for help.

Having said that, there are many ways in which herbs can work quickly and effectively, and this is the second level of action, that of first aid. When you wash a wound with an infusion of *Calendula* (marigold), for example, it sets to work immediately, discouraging infection and soothing inflammation. When a child is screaming with the pain of earache, a couple of drops of oil of *Lavandula vera* (lavender) in the affected ear can calm it down instantly. It is likely that the herbs in this book that I have chosen for their first-aid qualities will be the ones that you will turn to the most, and many of the others can also be used in this way.

We usually apply first aid ourselves, and it is only when self-help doesn't work that we call in the professionals. This used to be the case for infections as well, but today many mothers tend to take their children to the doctor every time the children develop a cold or sore throat. This is partly because we are better informed and, as a result of the enormous amount of media attention given to terrible diseases like meningitis, tend to fear the worst – which, indeed, does sometimes happen. But don't forget the

Washing a wound thoroughly.

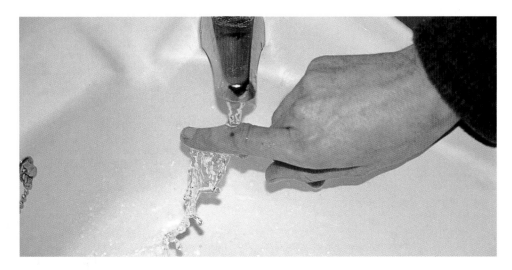

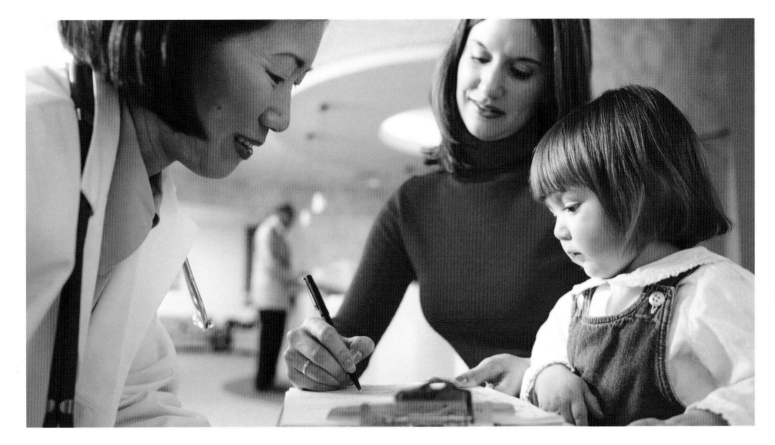

basic principle learned by all general practitioners early in their training: common things are common. In other words, your child is far more likely to have a simple cold than meningitis, and careful nursing is what is needed rather than medication.

These days, doctors are, in any case, more reluctant to prescribe antibiotics for every infection. We now understand their limitations and drawbacks better, and we know that their overuse simply leads to the emergence of drug-resistant organisms. However, not using them leaves a gap, and the doctor generally has nothing to offer as an alternative. I see a great many people, young and old, who are suffering from repeated infections, particularly ear infections, sinusitis, bronchitis, cystitis and thrush. Antibiotics will get rid of one infection, only for another to appear, and after a while both doctor and patient become wary of using them again. But what else can you do? In herbal terms, there are plenty of options.

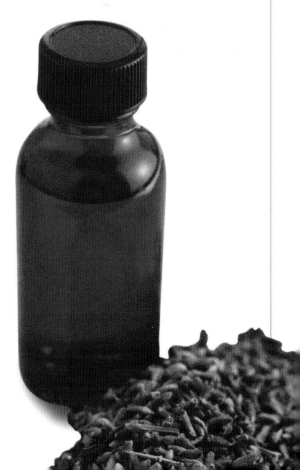

Lavender:
dried flowers and essential oil

The first thing is to try to work out why you are suffering from one infection after another. Unless your immunity has been compromised because of some genetic predisposition, the answer will nearly always be that stress is sapping your immunity. It could either be stress of a non-physical kind or something that you are doing that your body finds hard to cope with. Certain foods, particularly cows'-milk products and a range of food additives, can affect your immunity if you are sensitive to them, for instance. Some working environments offer a constant supply of infections, if you are vulnerable to them, air-conditioned offices and school classrooms being two obvious examples. Once you have identified any likely stress factors, you can then take steps either to avoid them or to minimize their effects on you as best you can.

The other option is to become stronger so that you are less open to infection. We all need to learn how to manage stress as we go through life, and there are a number of tried-and-true antidotes. Regular exercise, for example, especially vigorous aerobic movement, is beneficial in almost every way – indeed, its positive effects cannot be overestimated. Meditation is a touchstone for many people, enabling them to step away from their everyday concerns for a while. And the learning of life skills, so that you can hold your own and deal with whatever comes your way, is something that never stops as long as you live. If the coping mechanisms that you learned as a child or young adult

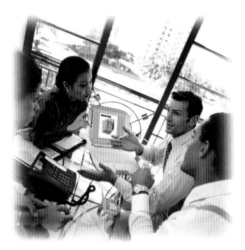

The office – a good place to catch a cold.

are not serving you very well today, remember that counseling and a host of other techniques can help you to learn new ones.

On the physical level, you can maintain the health of your immune system by eating plenty of fresh fruit, vegetables and polyunsaturated fats, and cutting down on saturated fats and processed foods. You can also augment a healthy diet with herbs. While some, like *Echinacea spp.* (coneflower), stimulate the immune function directly, others support its work by boosting the circulation (*Achillea millefolium*, or yarrow, for example) and the lymphatic system (*Galium aparine*, cleavers or goosegrass) or by helping to deal with inflammation (such as *Glycyrrhiza*

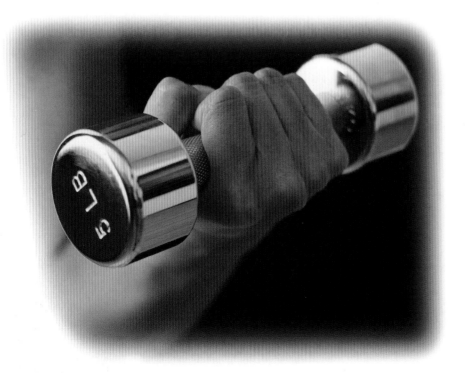

Strengthening exercises help boost the immune system.

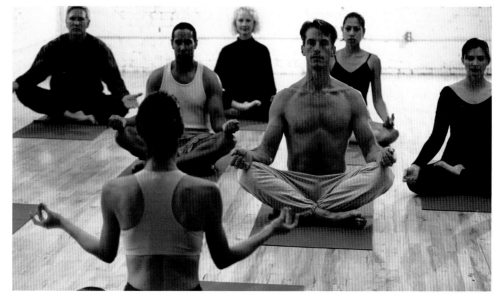

glabra, or licorice). Some, like *Solidago virgaurea,* or goldenrod, act as a tonic for the mucus membranes of the respiratory tract and urinary system, while yet others improve your ability to cope with stress (good examples are *Passiflora incarnata*, passionflower, or *Hypericum perforatum*, St. John's Wort). With all of these strategies in place, things should only get better, but if they don't, it's time to seek professional help. Yet even a deeply entrenched pattern of chronic ill health can respond to herbal medicine, and this applies as much to auto-immune problems as to acute infections. There is a whole range of conditions that come under the auto-immune heading, from rheumatoid

Regular yoga sessions can help you cope with stress.

arthritis to some types of thyroid disease. What they all have in common is that – for reasons that are not always clear – the body's immune defenses have turned against themselves. Once this happens, it is very difficult to halt the process: it is as though the body has entered into a state of panic and can no longer listen to the voice of reason. Nevertheless, herbs can help. It may appear contradictory to use an immune-system-stimulating herb like *Echinacea* (coneflower) when the immune system is already hyperactive, but because its action is restorative, it will tend to encourage the re-establishment of normal functions.

Thus, if your immune system's responses are depressed, *Echinacea* (coneflower) will cause them to become more active, but if they are overactive, they will be calmed down.

All in all, it is usually possible to use herbs to ease the situation in some way, perhaps by working in conjunction with orthodox drugs or other forms of therapy. Again, however, we are now moving beyond self-help into the realm of the professional herbalist.

49

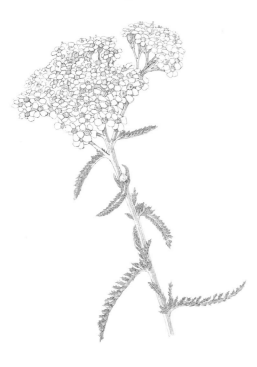

Fresh fruit boosts immunity.

Achillea millefolium (yarrow)

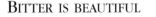
BITTER IS BEAUTIFUL

This section could equally have been called "If it tastes bad, it must be good for you." Strangely enough, there is more than a grain of truth in this. Many herbal remedies are bitter, and while the bitterness of some, such as *Cichorium intybus* (chicory) or *Taraxacum officinalis* (dandelion), is mild enough to make them fairly palatable, others, like *Artemisia absinthium* (wormwood) are positively tongue-shriveling. Although we generally tend to avoid bitter tastes, in small amounts bitterness has a very valuable role to play.

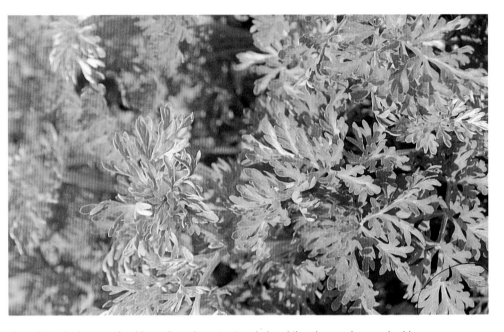

Some bitter herbs are palatable, and can be eaten in salads, while others make you shudder.

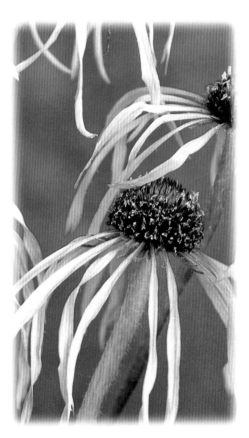

Echinacea angustifolia (coneflower) stimulates the immune system.

If you hold a drop of something bitter – tincture of *Taraxacum officinale radix* (dandelion root), perhaps – in your mouth for a minute, besides making you shudder, you will notice that it makes your saliva start to flow. Because bitterness is an irritant, saliva is produced to dilute it and wash it away. But the digestive system operates a kind of telegraph system so that it can react appropriately to food in the mouth, so the wake-up call caused by the bitter taste is passed on, from the mouth to the stomach and from there to the small intestine and colon. Along the way, digestive juices begin to flow. Bitterness stimulates the release of bile from the gall bladder in particular, which in turn improves the drainage of the liver.

Bitter remedies therefore improve our digestion, enabling our bodies to make better use of the food that we eat. They sharpen the appetite, restoring enjoyment of food to people who are run-down, convalescent or even anorexic. They also make you more aware of what you are eating and help you to judge whether or not you're really enjoying it, thus giving you an opportunity to shake off bad habits like eating too much or eating the wrong things. By stimulating the liver, bitter herbs do even more, however.

The liver governs almost everything that occurs within the body, from the absorption and storage of nutrients to the breakdown of toxins; and from the regulation of hormones to immunity and allergic responses. As a rule, if

The liver: powerhouse of the body.

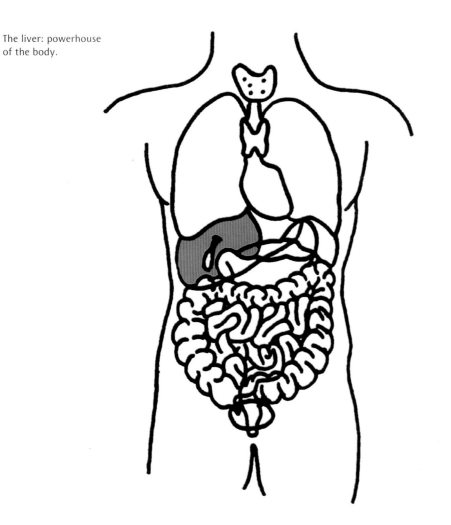

the liver is working well and everything is running smoothly, there shouldn't be much wrong anywhere else within the body. If it is not working properly, however, it can give rise to all sorts of symptoms, from feeling irritable to constipation, headaches, and tiredness, to more serious conditions like auto-immune problems, e.g. rheumatoid arthritis. Many side effects imposed by various drugs arise not just from their direct action within the body, but also from the extra burden that they place on the liver. These effects can be minimized or avoided altogether if you take some liver-supporting herbs like *Taraxacum officinale radix* (dandelion root) or *Carduus marianus* (blessed thistle) alongside your drug regime.

A bitter aperitif will help you digest a rich feast.

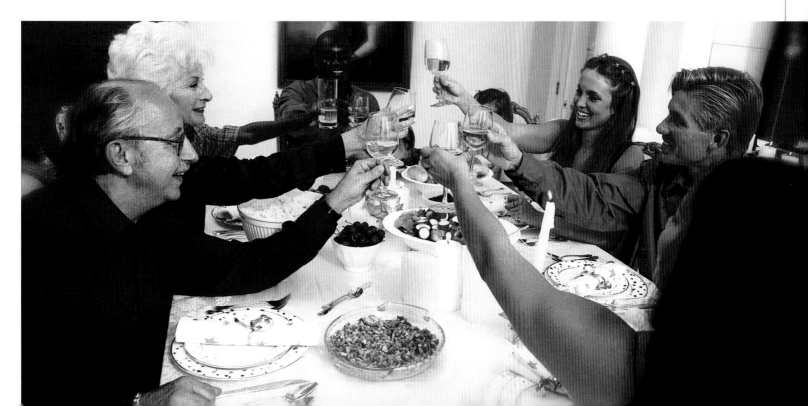

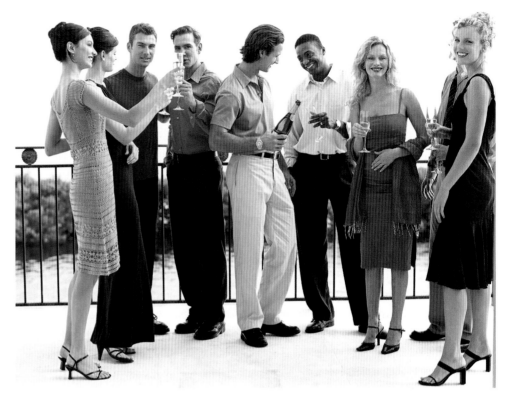

THE DIGESTIVE SYSTEM

The digestive system is basically a tube, some 33 feet/eleven meters long, which stretches (or rather coils) between the mouth and the anus. Because its surfaces are a modified form of skin, many herbs that are beneficial to the skin will also help to heal the gut. Its function is to bring the outside inside: to enable us to absorb nutrients but not too many of the sub-

Herbs may help the "morning after" feeling.

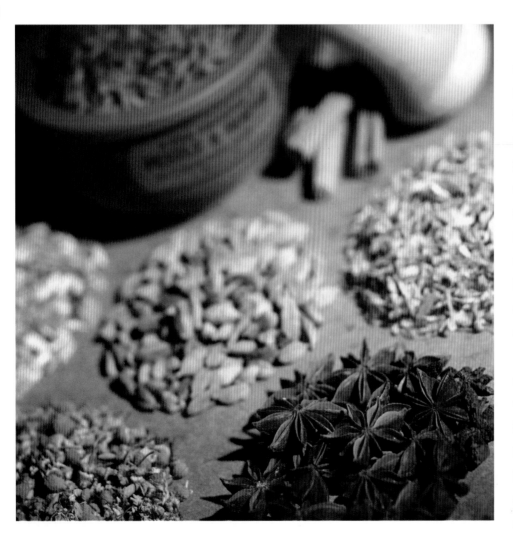

Herbs can stimulate digestion, leading to a healthier life.

stances that could harm us. The digestive system is highly sophisticated, but not foolproof. When it is working efficiently, you will be almost entirely unaware of anything that occurs between swallowing your food and passing motions. When it is not, however, symptoms such as cramping pain, gas, bloating, vomiting, diarrhea and constipation can make you feel extremely uncomfortable.

With their food-like quality, herbs are in their element when working within the digestive system. A diet that is rich in herbs and spices will go a long way toward ensuring good health. As well as tasting delicious, these herbs stimulate your digestion, discourage parasites and other unfriendly organisms from taking hold and generally keep the digestive system on its toes. Most of the herbs that are commonly added to food are essentially warming, which means that the only time when they are not of help is when the digestive system is already overheated, perhaps caused by conditions such as stomach ulcers and some bowel problems. In such cases, bland food is required to avoid further irritation, while cooling, soothing remedies like *Symphytum officinale* (comfrey), *Althaea officinalis* (marshmallow root) and *Ulmus fulva* (slippery elm bark) may also be useful.

The key to using herbs effectively is to think in terms of balance: which way has the balance tipped, and what would help to restore its equilibrium?

I shall now work through the components of the digestive system, looking at some common problems and what may cause them, and suggesting the herbs that may help to alleviate those symptoms. Again, the golden rule is to try them out and, if they haven't helped within a reasonable time, to seek professional guidance.

Comfrey (*symphytum*): soothes upset stomachs.

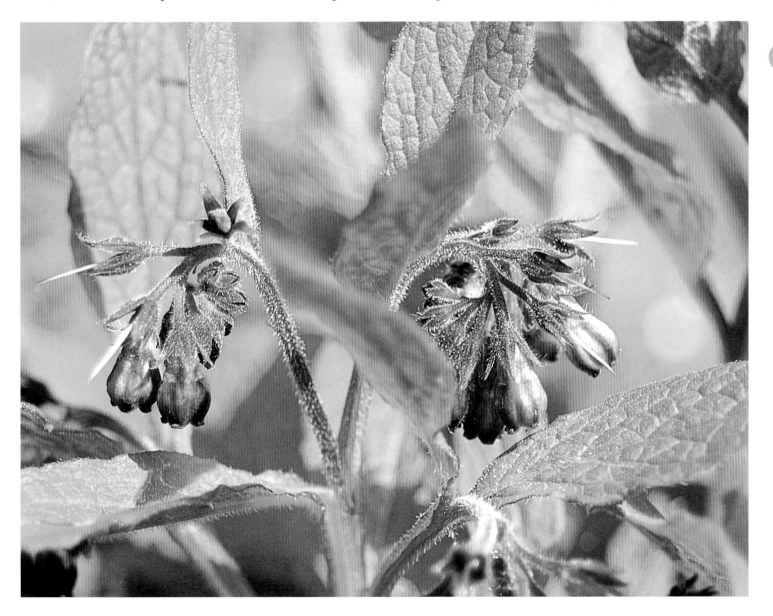

53

Ginger root aids digestion.

like *Calendula* (marigold) and *Salvia* (sage). It may also be advisable to use a softer toothbrush or to brush your teeth and gums less vigorously.

Once you have them, cold sores tend to recur, particularly when you are run-down. A mouthwash of *Salvia* (sage) will help an outbreak to clear up faster, while taking *Echinacea* (coneflower) can keep your mouth symptom-free for longer periods than usual.

The stomach

The stomach is essentially a bath of acid that is designed to begin the breakdown of food and to kill anything living that you have swallowed before it descends dangerously far. Trouble starts when acid leaks out of the stomach into the gullet or small intestine (neither of which are designed to withstand it), or when the stomach lining itself is damaged. Stress and anxiety tend to result in more acid being produced, which increases the likelihood of developing gastritis and ulcers. Smoking, along with some foods, notably red meat and saturated fats, also increases the

production of stomach acid. By contrast, insufficient acid may be produced if the digestive system becomes run-down, creating a vicious circle that is particularly common among elderly people, who often eat fewer and fewer stimulating foods, their stomachs thus becoming less able to cope with them.

Good teeth are the first step to good digestion.

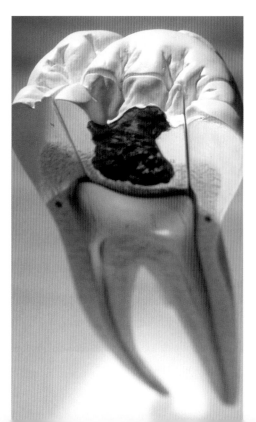

Oil of cloves is good for alleviating toothache.

The mouth

Toothache, of course, requires the attention of a dentist, although using the traditional herbal remedy, oil of cloves (*Caryophyllum*), will help to ease the pain.

Gum problems, such as bleeding gums and gingivitis, respond well to astringent, anti-inflammatory herbs

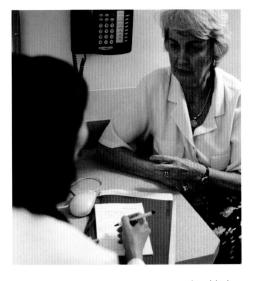

For stomach problems caused by anxiety, try *Matricaria* (chamomile) and *Melissa* (lemon balm).

For too much stomach acid, use *Filipendula* (meadowsweet); for too little, mild bitters like *Verbena* (vervain).

For ulcers and gastritis, long-term treatment will be needed, not only because the symptoms can disappear for a while and then flare up again, but because it takes long time for the stomach lining to heal. Soothing, protective herbs like *Symphytum* (comfrey), *Glycyrrhiza* (licorice), *Calendula* (marigold) and *Althaea* officinalis (marshmallow root) should be of help.

For gas (belching), try teas made with *Mentha piperita* (peppermint), *Melissa* (lemon balm) or *Foeniculum vulgare* (fennel). Also ask yourself whether you are either eating foods that your stomach is not happy with or are leaving it too long before eating after you've suffered your first hunger pangs.

For nausea, any of the bitter herbs

Digestive troubles are common among the elderly.

may help. *Zingiber* (ginger) and *Mentha piperita* (peppermint) are tried-and-tested remedies, too.

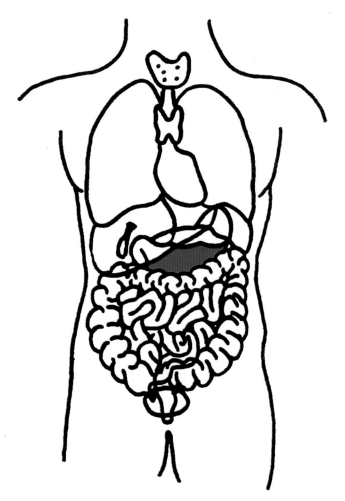

The stomach

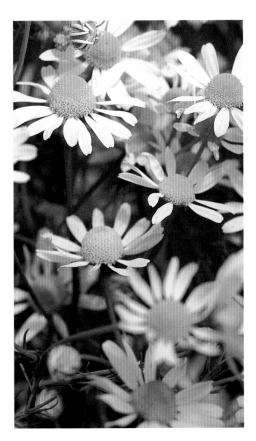

Chamomile (*Matricaria*) soothes the stomach.

The small intestine

Because the absorption of nutrients takes place within the small intestine, if it is diseased, there is a strong case for using vitamin and mineral supplements to ensure that your nutritional status doesn't become compromised.

The two most common disease processes that affect the small intestine are ulcerative colitis and Crohn's disease. Both result in ulceration and inflammation, and the same herbs that work on the stomach will do good here. Treating them is definitely a long-term job, however, and because relapses can be triggered even when there have been no symptoms for years, sufferers must stay vigilant. When the problem is acute, fasting (but only with the guidance of a professional) may be the only way to calm the inflammation down because the constant passage of food through the gut will irritatate the inflamed patches over again.

Another problem that can affect the small intestine is difficulty in breaking down certain foods, resulting in gas and bloating, as the smooth movement of the gut is interrupted. The two most likely culprits are dairy products and wheat, both of which contain very large proteins. According to one theory, these proteins can actually damage the gut lining both in

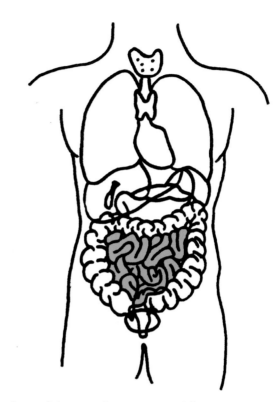

Small intestine

babies who are given dairy products or wheat before their digestive systems are able to cope with them, and in susceptible individuals of all ages. The consequence may be a "leaky gut," enabling certain unwelcome substances to pass through the damaged membrane to cause a variety of

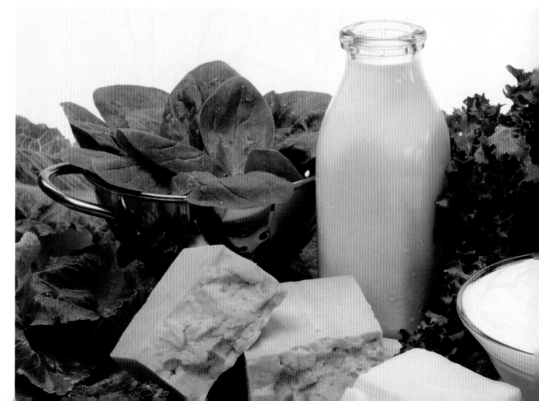

56

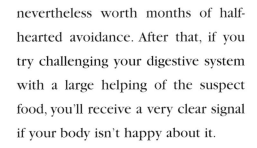

problems. Although I am not sure how sound this theory actually is, I do know that removing wheat or dairy products – or both – from the diet for a time, as well as taking herbs like *Symphytum* (comfrey), *Calendula* (marigold) and *Foeniculum vulgare* (fennel), to name just a few, can bring about a huge improvement. Again, it is best to undertake this with the help of a herbalist, and to do it wholeheartedly. You will have to abstain totally from the suspect foods, otherwise nothing will be proved, and because most of us eat dairy products and wheat in some form every day, cutting them out of your diet will take careful planning. A week of complete abstention is

Calcium-rich foods

nevertheless worth months of half-hearted avoidance. After that, if you try challenging your digestive system with a large helping of the suspect food, you'll receive a very clear signal if your body isn't happy about it.

People with a food intolerance often worry that they will have to avoid their problem foods for the rest of their lives. Not so, in my experience: if you stay away from them for a while, and at the same time strengthen your digestive system with herbs, you should be able to eat them from time to time. Just how long it will take you to build up your tolerance to varies from person to person, and you will only know how your body will respond to them if you take the risk of trying them now and again. But, if you

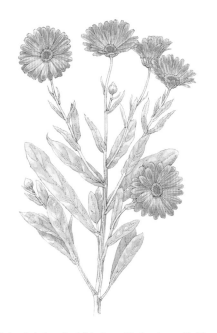

Calendula (marigold) helps with food sensitivities.

resume eating a lot of your problem food, the intolerance is likely to flare up again. Everyone is different, and it is up to you to learn your own limits.

Fennel (*Foeniculum vulgare*) soothes gut tension.

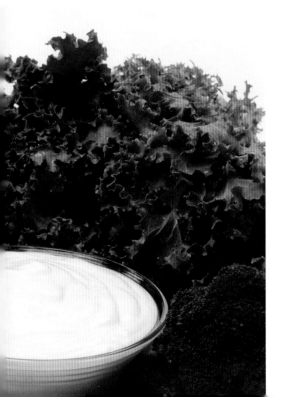

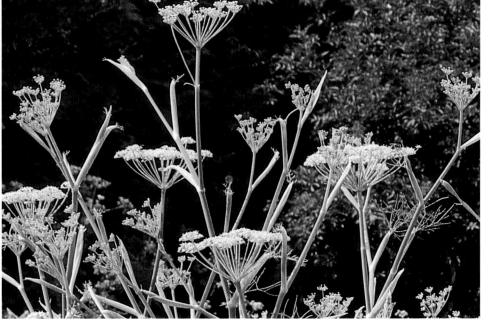

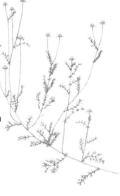

Matricaria (chamomile)soothes an irritable bowel.

The large intestine

Some absorption occurs within the large intestine, mainly of water. If all goes well, by the time what remains of the food that you've eaten reaches the last part of its journey, it will have been transformed into firm stools that are evacuated regularly. All sorts of things can happen to upset this process, however. Everyone has occasional bouts of gas, stomach pain, constipation or diarrhea, and usually we recover within a few days, but if the problem continues, we start to use labels like "irritable bowel syndrome" and, in older people, "diverticular disease." These things are so common

Hops are calming for the gut.

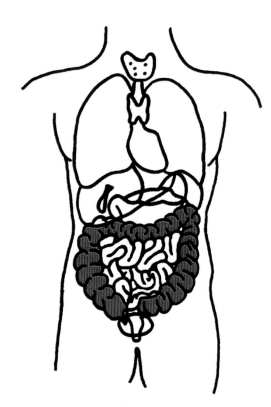

Large Intestine.

as to be almost normal, but they can be miserable to live with, so what can we do to alleviate them?

The damage may have started with an infection, which, although it may have cleared up long ago, has left a residue of scarring and inflammation that, once it has become chronic, is very hard to shift. Food intolerances play their part, too. Anxiety is also renowned for its bowel-disrupting effects and, again, once a habit has been formed, it can be very stubborn. The same herbs that are employed higher up the digestive tract can be useful here because their actions are just as valuable within the colon. They include *Symphytum* (comfrey) to soothe, *Melissa* (lemon balm) or

Matricaria (chamomile) to ease spasms and acute stomach pain, *Allium sativum* (garlic) to help to clear up infections and *Valeriana officinalis* (valerian) or *Humulus lupulus* (hop) for anxiety.

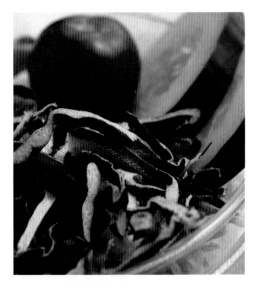

Fresh vegetables keep your system moving.

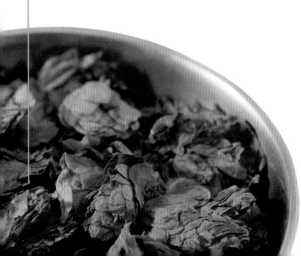

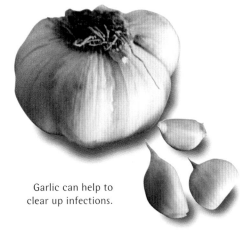

Garlic can help to clear up infections.

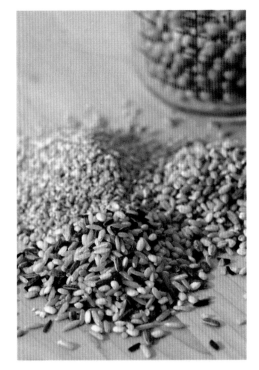

Rice: a food that is gentle on the system.

When the bowel is in a really excitable state, however, taking anything at all (including food) will make the symptoms worse. In this case, the large intestine needs very careful, gentle treatment, including fasting and soothing remedies. The orthodox medical wisdom recommends a high-fiber diet for an irritable bowel, but there is fiber and then there is fiber. Wheat bran, which is what people often turn to, is particularly scratchy, which is the last thing your tender, inflamed tissues need – it's a little like scouring a patch of sunburned skin with steel wool. Soft vegetable fiber is what is required, and the best source of this is root vegetables. Although you should avoid wheat, other cereals, such as rice (without the husks), and oats should be fine and will give your poor, tortured bowel the equivalent of a gentle massage.

For treating constipation, too, bulk vegetable fibers are much more effective than stimulating laxatives – even herbal ones – which bully and scourge the bowel into action, often causing a good deal of stomach pain. Such laxatives are also habit-forming, and once you start taking them, you'll find that you have to keep on doing so. Coming off laxatives is harder than weaning yourself off tranquilizers, in my experience, and people often choose not to try. If you do become constipated, and eating lots of fruit and vegetables hasn't helped, try bulk laxatives such as *Psyllium* (flea seed) or *Linum* (linseed) before resorting to the big guns. Bitters like *Taraxacum officinale radix* (dandelion root) or *Rumex crispus* (curled dock) can sometimes help too.

The last word goes to hemorrhoids, which are usually provoked either by straining when constipated or when pushing in childbirth. Although a soothing cream containing *Calendula* (marigold) or *Potentilla tormentilla* (tormentil) will relieve the soreness and itching, prevention lies in the management methods described above for constipation. Remember that once you've had hemorrhoids, any straining can set them off again, and in this case prevention is definitely better than cure!

Root vegetables: the best source of bulk fiber.

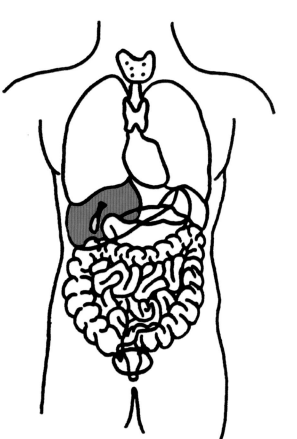

Liver/gall bladder.

60

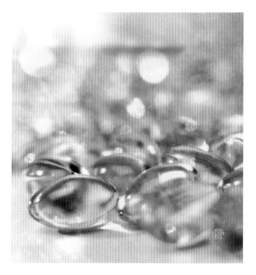

Garlic capsules can help support the digestion.

THE LIVER AND GALL BLADDER

The liver, which governs nearly everything that occurs within the body, secretes bile, a bitter substance that is stored in the gall bladder and released into the small intestine when food is on its way there. Because the particular function of bile is to break down fats, if the liver isn't secreting bile as it should, you won't be able to digest fatty foods very well. You will suffer from symptoms such as nausea, gas, bloating and diarrhea, as well as feeling "liverish," that is, irritable and out of sorts. If the gall bladder becomes inflamed or develops stones, the episodes of acute pain that result will leave you no alternative but to seek prompt medical help.

If the liver isn't happy, its many other functions will be disrupted, too. And, besides helping to break down food, it stores some nutrients, plays a large part in regulating the responses of the immune system and hormone levels, and breaks down toxins (including most orthodox drugs, as well as alcohol). But what makes the liver unhappy? First, infections, like hepatitis or glandular fever, which leave a shadow that can take months, or even years, to lift; second, being overloaded with toxins, such as alcohol, food additives and drugs; and, thirdly a diet that is too rich in saturated fats. The liver can cope with these last two burdens for a long time,

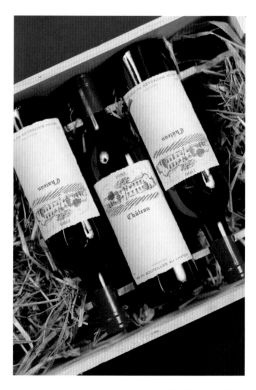

Too much wine and rich living can lead to trouble.

and it is often not until a person is in their forties that liver trouble – along with a mid-life crisis – starts to show. This is why restoring the liver's health can be a slow business: if it's taken a lifetime to get to this point, the trouble isn't going to clear up within a few weeks.

The good news, however, is that when you start taking bitter herbs like *Taraxacum* (dandelion), *Verbena* (vervain) and *Rumex crispus* (curled dock) you may start to feel better almost immediately. All of these help to kick-start the liver into action and you can take them for as long as you like. I've had many patients who've had their gall bladders removed because of stones or inflammation, only to find that their digestive problems have not improved, and, indeed, have even, in some cases, become worse. I've found that it's always possible for them to improve their condition with bitter herbs, usually by taking at least a small dose continually for some months (and it's wise to have some on hand if you are planning a big feast). A small price to pay for relief from years of misery.

Dandelion root supports the liver.

Vervain (*Verbena officinalis*): a gentle bitter.

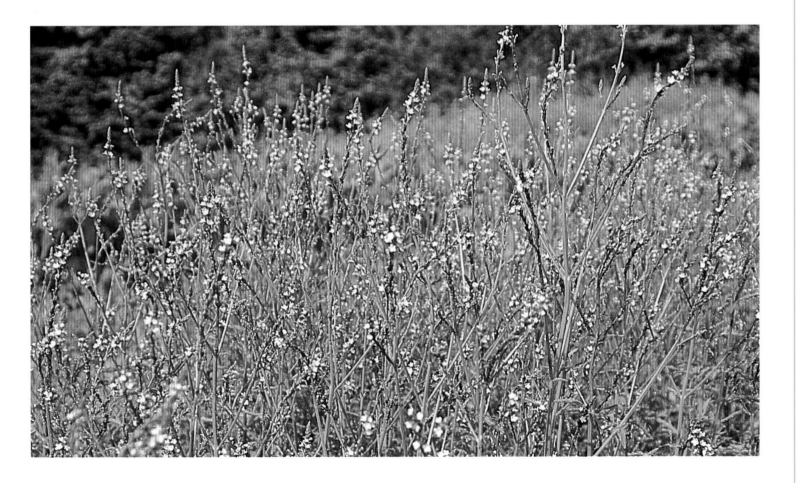

THE RESPIRATORY SYSTEM

There are two parts to the respiratory system: the upper part, which includes the ears, nose and throat, and the lower part, which consists of the lungs and bronchi. Both are lined with moist mucus membranes, which are designed to warm incoming air and to trap unwelcome particles and infectious organisms. They do this very efficiently, which is why the infection that we experience the most often is the common cold. It's not the cold itself that bothers us, it's the body's own efforts to deal with it. The mucus membranes become swollen and congested and lots of mucus is produced, which streams down the nose and throat and can become stuck in confined spaces like the sinuses and the Eustachian tube leading to the middle ear. You may also develop a fever and will certainly feel lousy for a few days.

When treating a cold, the problem can be that suppressing its symptoms simply prolongs the infection, sometimes also leaving you vulnerable to catching more colds. It's good to relieve congestion by encouraging the mucus to flow more freely, but it's not good to do this by suppressing it with decongestants, because although it will dry up, making you feel better for a few hours, the dam will then burst and the mucus will flood back again.

Similarly, it's acceptable to encourage your immune system to do its infection-fighting work (see "Feed a fever?" page 64), but not to try to prevent it from ever succumbing to an infection. This is because our bodies are designed to suffer acute illnesses from time to time, and there

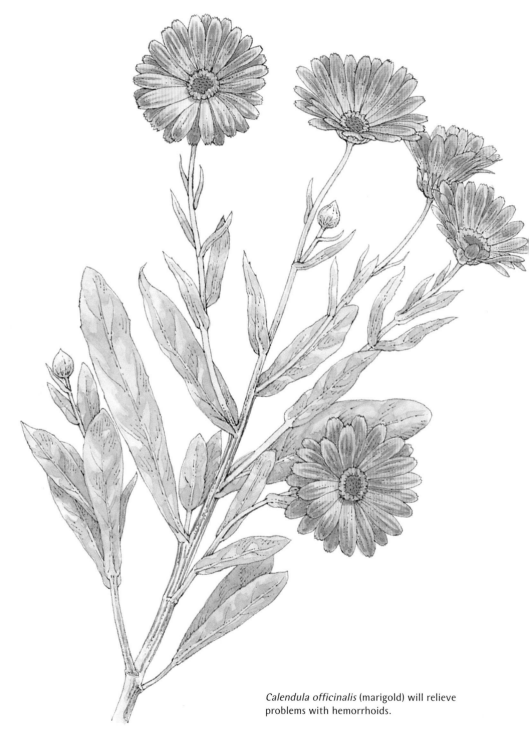

Calendula officinalis (marigold) will relieve problems with hemorrhoids.

62

is growing suspicion within medical circles that not allowing that to happen may pave the way for more serious problems later on. In other words, if the immune system never has a workout, it may not be able to respond properly when you really need it to and may also start responding to the wrong things, leading to allergy problems and auto-immune diseases. It's therefore best to give in to a respiratory infection gracefully.

You should only suppress a cold or flu in someone whose vitality is too low to deal with it. For example, a child in danger of convulsions, or a person on immuno-suppressive drugs or whose immunity has been compromised by a disease such as AIDS, or an elderly person whose life force is dwindling.

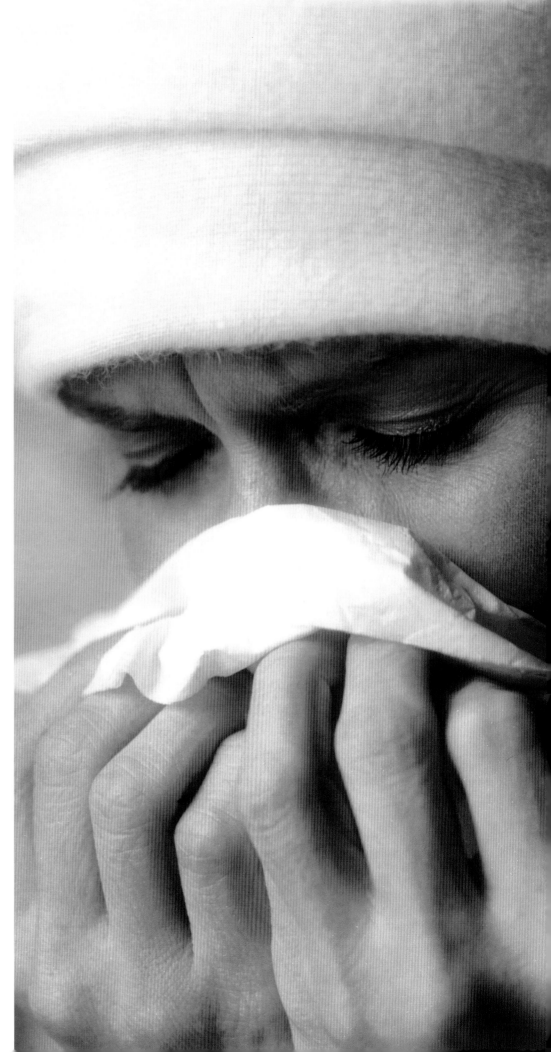

Catching a cold is not always a bad thing.

FEED A FEVER

Have you got a chill? Are you feeling shivery and achy and think that you're starting a bout of flu or a bad cold? If so, take some aspirin and your temperature will come down and consequently you'll feel better. So says conventional wisdom. However, it pays to look at the reason for the fever before you dampen down the fire.

In fact, it's not the flu or the stomach upset that gives you the fever, it's your own immune system going into action on your behalf. As your core temperature rises, your defenses become more lively, diverting attention from the normal activities of a healthy body – eating and digesting food and running around getting on with your life – so that all you want to do is to crawl into bed. This is exactly as it should be: once there, you'll cook up a good sweat and your body will get on with the business of repelling the invading organisms, which, in turn, will become more unhappy and reproduce more slowly as the battle heats

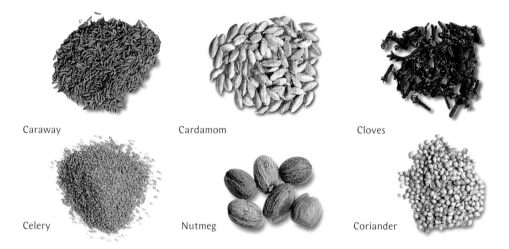

Caraway   Cardamom   Cloves

Celery   Nutmeg   Coriander

up. If, on the other hand, you swallow the aspirin and struggle on heroically, the defensive process is suppressed. Add antibiotics to the aspirin, and you'll smother the flames even further: although the antibiotics may kill the bacteria, they'll do nothing for your infected tissues because they'll

suppress your system's ability to do its important defensive work. If you're basically healthy and vigorous, you'll shake off the infection eventually, but it may take a little longer than it would have if you hadn't taken antibiotics, and it's likely that you won't feel up to scratch for some time afterward, too.

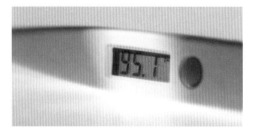

Temperatures can vary as your body fights a fever.

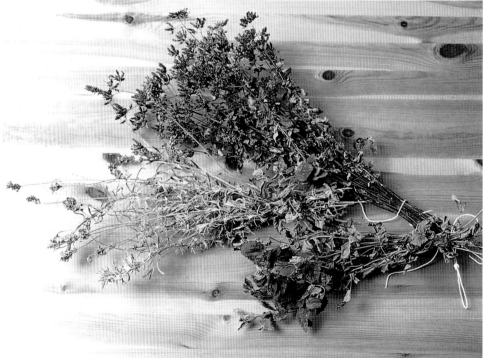

Herb teas will help you to have a good illness.

A fever should therefore be welcomed as a sign that your immune system is in vigorous form. That having been said, if your temperature rises too high or lasts for too long, it will take its toll, and fevers in the very young, the very old or people whose immune systems have been compromised must be nursed with special care. In general, however, if you can afford the luxury of going straight to bed for a day or two, you'll emerge feeling refreshed, and maybe even better than you felt before. If you manage it well, an episode of acute illness can cleanse your system and can also help you to throw off longer-term problems, such as niggling phlegm, aching joints and low energy levels.

For these reasons, it's worth thinking twice before trying to knock a fever on the head. Instead, try taking herbs that support the body's defensive efforts: remedies like *Allium sativum* (garlic), *Echinacea* (coneflower), *Achillea millefolium* (yarrow) and the flowers of *Sambucus nigra* (elder). Then go to bed, drink plenty and eat sparingly. Your colleagues will thank you for not bringingt your bugs to work, and you health will benefit from having gone through an ultimately restorative illness.

Colds and flu

Some foods, notably dairy products and fatty foods, tend both to encourage mucus formation and to make it stickier. If you have trouble with phlegm and are constantly blowing your nose or clearing your throat, it's worth either reducing the amount of these foods that you eat or cutting them out of your diet altogether. If you are prone to colds, sinusitis, ear infections or chest infections, this strategy should be doubly helpful. And even if you only catch the occasional cold, it will be shorter and less messy if you cut out milk from your diet for a few days.

Your intake of the foods that encourage the flow of mucus and make it more liquid, on the other hand, should be increased. These include fruits of all sorts and the Allium family of vegetables, which includes onions, garlic, shallots, spring onions and chives.

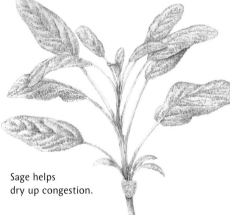

Cow's milk can cause problems.

To relieve the misery of a cold, you'll probably find a tea made with *Sambucus* (elder), *Achillea* (yarrow) and *Mentha piperita* (peppermint) very comforting. A hot drink made with lemon and honey is a well-known cold remedy, and you can give it some extra bite with a pinch of cin-

Eucalyptus oil can help clear blocked sinuses.

Sage helps dry up congestion.

65

namon, cloves, coriander or ginger. Herbs that are good to mix with hot water to inhale include *Eucalyptus globulus* (eucalyptus), *Thymus vulgaris* (thyme), *Pinus sylvestris* (pine) and *Mentha piperita* (peppermint). Taking *Echinacea* (coneflower) and *Allium sativum* (garlic) will support your immune system as it goes to work. Other than that, the key to treating a cold so that you'll bounce back to health after two or three days is good nursing, eating lightly and resting.

Following a debilitating dose of flu, *Verbena officinalis* (vervain) or I*nula helenium* (elecampane) will help the patient's convalescence.

Oil of lavender is an excellent first aid for earache.

Ear problems

Middle-ear infections can be painful and persistent because the Eustachian tubes are very narrow and easily blocked. I see a lot of children (and some adults) who have been repeatedly treated with antibiotics, only to develop ear infections. Now that tubes have fallen from favor, medicine is stuck for solutions, but there remain plenty of herbs that will gently tone the congested membranes and get the mucus moving again. Try mucus-membrane tonics like *Plantago lanceolata* (ribwort), *Verbascum thapsus* (mullein) or *Solidago virgaurea* (goldenrod), together with any of the remedies

Making a hot lemon drink.

mentioned above for treating colds and flu. It may take some time, but even the most stubborn infection will shift from the ear in the end (and the response is much faster in children than in adults).

For earache, introducing a drop or two of *Lavandula vera* (lavender) oil in the ear will help immediately.

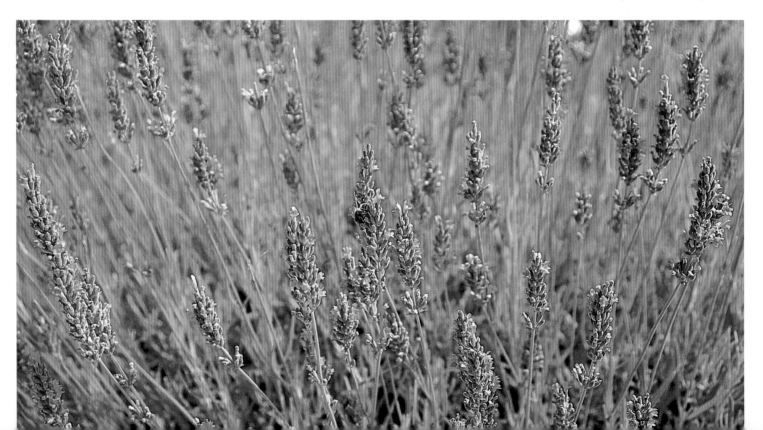

Hay fever (allergic rhinitis)

Hay fever responds well to herbs, and, although you may have to take a lot of them at first, the amount you need will usually fall as time goes on. Ideally you should start to take herbs a month or so before the hay fever season begins, but they do a good first-aid job as well. Try *Plantago* (ribwort), *Urtica dioca* (nettle), *Sambucus* (elder) and *Euphrasia* (eyebright). If hay fever makes your eyes sore, an eyewash made from *Matricaria* (chamomile) or *Euphrasia* (eyebright), or both, will usually bring quick relief. There are stronger remedies, too, but these are only available from herbal practitioners because their dosage needs to be carefully controlled.

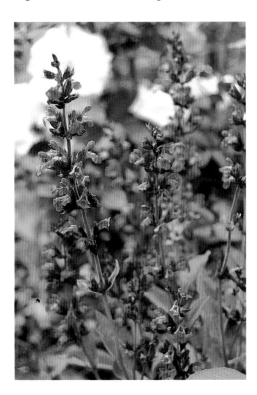

Sage (*Salvia officinalis*): soothing for sore throats.

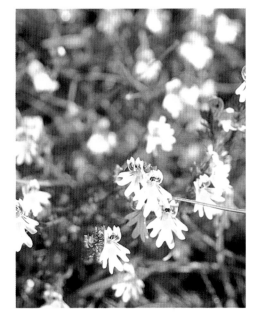

Eyebright (*Euphrasia*) helps hay fever symptoms.

Sore throats

To clear up the infection and calm the inflammation caused by a sore throat, tonsilitis, laryngitis or pharyngitis, use *Salvia officinalis* (sage), *Calendula officinalis* (marigold) or *Thymus vulgaris (thyme)*. Add some *Galium aparine* (cleavers or goosegrass) if the lymph glands need to be cleared.

Coughs

A persistent cough will respond, in time, to any of the herbs mentioned above for treating colds and flu because they address the cause of the irritation. What you must not do, however, is to suppress a cough – after all, it has developed for the purpose of clearing mucus from the chest. If the

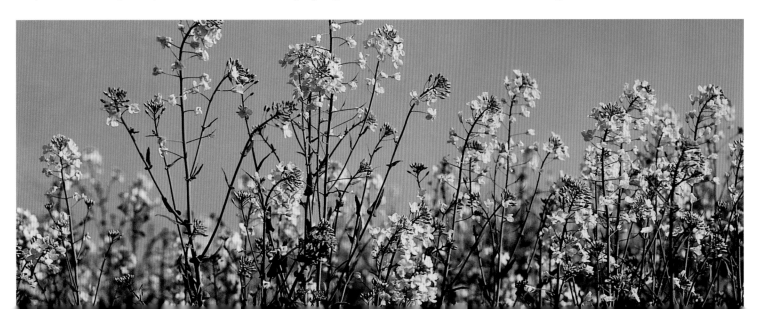

The pollen season brings misery to some.

Yoga helps to keep the lungs clear.

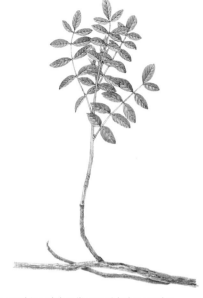

Glycyrrhiza glabra (licorice) helps resolve chest infections.

An essential oil burner works while you sleep.

cough is unproductive, on the other hand, and is waking you (and perhaps your bedfellow) at night and wearing you down, the inflammation will need stronger measures to send it on its way. *Symphytum* (comfrey) and *Althaea radix* (marshmallow or hollyhock) are soothing herbs, while *Glycyrrhiza* (licorice), *Thymus* (thyme) and *Inula helenium* (elecampane) are also anti-inflammatory. If you are really desperate for a few hours free of coughing, *Prunus serotina* (wild cherry bark) will temporarily switch off the cough reflex.

Bronchitis and pneumonia

The anti-fever herbs (see "Feed a fever?", page 64) come into play when treating bronchitis and pneumonia, together with those that stimulate the flow of mucus: *Thymus* (thyme), *Inula* (elecampane) and *Symphytum* (comfrey) are especially useful. *Allium sativum* (garlic), however, is essential because it helps to disinfect the lungs from their bases upward, while *Echinacea* (coneflower) will work to fight the infection, too. Using inhalations and chest rubs, herbal baths and essential oil burners will also help. Regular breathing exercises may also be of enormous help (if they cause you to cough at first, so much the better). Yoga is excellent, too, and will help to speed up your recovery.

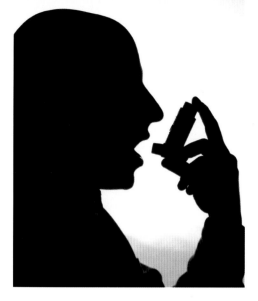

Using an inhaler to treat asthma.

Asthma

Unless your asthma is very mild, you will usually be relying on inhalers, but you may be able to reduce, or even eliminate, their use with herbs. Breathing exercises will also be a big help in managing asthma.

Asthma-aggravating infections require prompt treatment, but you can help to ward them off by taking *Allium sativum* (garlic) or *Echinacea* (coneflower) regularly. Besides the herbs that have already been mentioned in this respiratory-tract section, those that soothe anxiety, such as *Matricaria* (chamomile) or *Humulus lupulus* (hop), can be very useful. You can also get a prescription for stronger anti-spasmodic and anti-allergy herbs from a qualified herbalist.

As a first-aid measure when you feel an attack threatening, sniffing the essential oil of *Achillea* (yarrow) can sometimes either head it off or lessen its severity, so keep a bottle in your pocket or purse for emergencies.

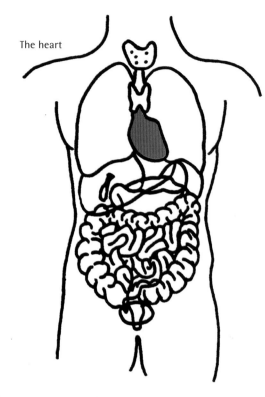

The heart

THE HEART AND CIRCULATION

The blood vessels are the body's transport system, taking food and oxygen to cells and carrying away waste products. If they are not doing their job well, everything else is affected, meaning you can nearly always improve a physical problem simply by supporting the circulation. The heart, which is the driving force behind it all, needs looking after, too. Regular exercise, both moderate and vigorous, will keep the heart healthy, as will a diet low in saturated fats and salt, moderate alcohol intake, no tobacco and effective stress management. You can also do a great deal with herbs.

There are a number of herbs to choose from for improving poor circulation. *Tilia* (lime flower), *Achillea* (yarrow), *Allium sativum* (garlic), *Zingiber* (ginger), *Rosmarinus officinalis* (rosemary) and *Ginkgo biloba* (ginkgo) are lead-

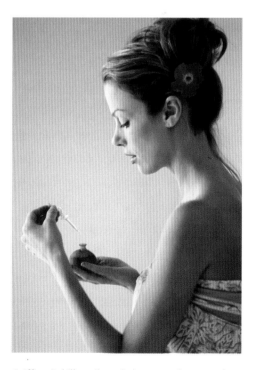

Sniffing Achillea oil can help ease asthma attacks.

69

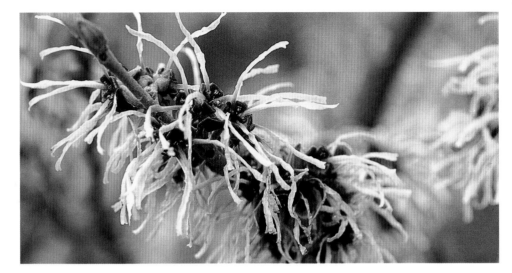

Witch hazel helps heal varicose veins.

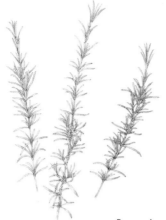

Rosmarinus officinalis
(rosemary) stimulates the circulation.

ers in the field, so try them all and see which ones suit you best. For cold hands and feet, including chilblains and Raynaud's disease, *Capsicum minimum* (cayenne) is useful, either taken internally (in small doses) or as a cream applied to the skin.

For varicose veins, try the herbs listed above, along with *Crataegus* (hawthorn) and *Aesculus hippocastanum* (horse chestnut), both of which help to tone the blood vessels' walls. For varicose eczema or phlebitis, use *Calendula* (marigold), *Symphytum* (comfrey) and *Oenothera* (evening primrose oil). For an external treatment, applying a lotion or compress made with *Calendula* (marigold), *Symphytum* (comfrey) and *Hamamelis virginiana* (witch hazel) will help. Even varicose ulcers can be healed, but

expert advice may be needed for this.

For the heart, *Crataegus* (hawthorn) is always appropriate, depending on the situation, perhaps backed up by other herbs. If anxiety is a factor, or the depression that can descend after a heart attack, use *Tilia* (lime flower), *Melissa* (lemon balm), *Valeriana* (valerian) or *Leonurus cardiaca* (mother- wort). If a diuretic is needed, the leaves of *Taraxacum officinale* (dandelion) will help,

although it is likely that drugs will be required too.

For high blood pressure, try *Crataegus* (hawthorn) with *Tilia* (lime flower) and *Achillea* (yarrow). Low blood pressure is only a problem if you tend to faint when you stand up suddenly, but it can indicate some debility, in which case try *Avena sativa* (oat straw) and *Verbena officinalis* (vervain).

Blood pressure can be managed with herbs.

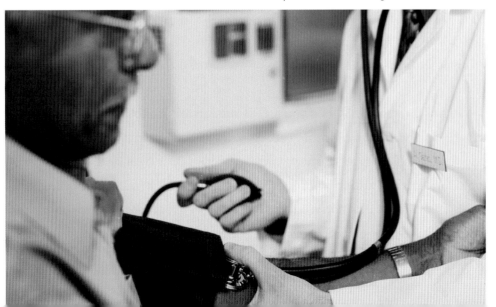

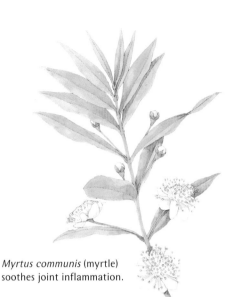

THE BONES AND MUSCLES

Most of the problems affecting the bones or muscles that you may want to treat will either be due to injuries or to internal processes such as rheumatoid and osteo-arthritis, all of which tend to involve the muscles, tendons, ligaments and joints rather than the bones themselves. In any case, the first thing to do is to support the circulation with herbs like *Achillea* (yarrow) and *Tilia* (lime flower) because the products of inflammation will need to be carried away to be replaced with a fresh supply of blood.

Two conditions that do affect the bones are fractures and osteoporosis, both of which can be helped by herbs that directly stimulate the bone-building process, *Symphytum* (comfrey), for instance, stimulating new cell growth and *Equisetum arvense* (horsetail) helping to replace lost calcium. Osteoporosis is a complex condition, and many factors may be involved. Doing weight-bearing exercise is crucial to keep on stimulating new bone growth, while herbs that give hormonal support may help, too:

Myrtus communis (myrtle) soothes joint inflammation.

Angelica sinensis (Chinese angelica or dong quai) and *Vitex agnus-castus* (chasteberry) are worth trying. Even if your doctor prescribes hormone replacement therapy (HRT), you can

Horsetail (*Equisetum*) helps to build strong bones.

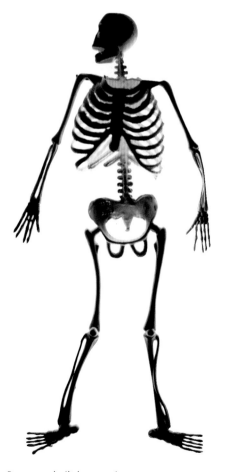

Bones are built by exercise.

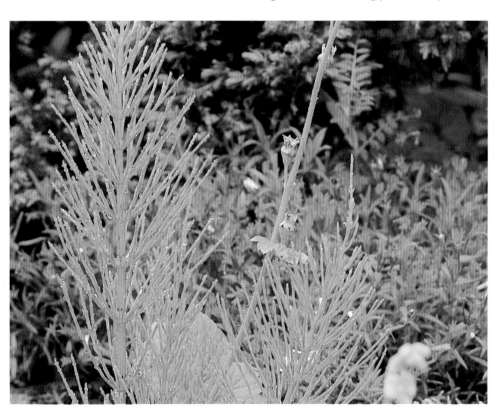

71

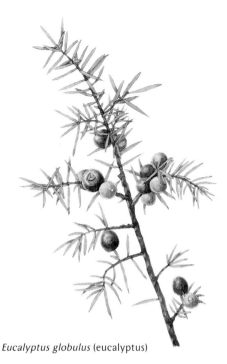

Eucalyptus globulus (eucalyptus)

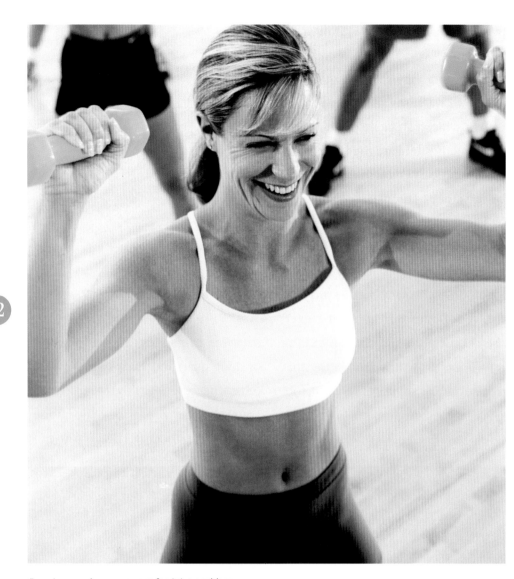

Exercise: good management for joint problems.

still use herbs to back it up and to buffer any unwanted side effects.

Besides providing circulatory support for strains and sprains, you can speed up healing with *Symphytum* (comfrey) and reduce inflammation with *Filipendula* (meadowsweet) and *Salix nigra* (willow bark). The same sort of management applies to osteo-arthritis, which is essentially a condition of wear and tear that affects certain joints. Although you can't reverse the damage, you can manage it and try to prevent it from becoming worse. Besides herbs, regular physical therapy – like massage, physiotherapy or gentle manipulation – is enormously helpful in maintaining mobility and reducing pain. For external treatment, there are plenty of warming herbs that will work to ease a sore joint, such as a cream with *Symphytum* (comfrey) as a base, along with the essential oils of, for example, *Juniperus communis* (juniper), *Myrtus communis* (myrtle), *Rosmarinus officinalis* (rosemary) or *Piper nigrum* (black pepper).

Rheumatoid arthritis, on the other hand, is a much more inflammatory condition than osteo-arthritis, and may start at a much earlier age, but it can be improved, or even completely cleared up, with good management. It is always worth investigating your diet to ascertain whether there are any irritants that could be avoided. The most likely culprits include wheat and dairy products, but perhaps also oranges, tomatoes, red meat, shellfish, peanuts (including peanut butter) and gout-aggravating foods that are rich in

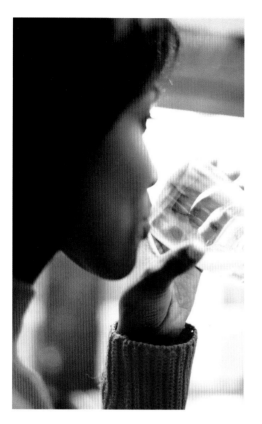

Fasting cleanses the system.

oxalic acid, such as spinach and strawberries. Coffee, tea and alcohol, especially red wine, can also worsen rheumatoid arthritis. If you suffer from this condition, I would strongly recommend that you undertake a fast – under professional supervision, of course – both to cleanse the system and, after you've started reintroducing the suspect foods into your diet one at a time, to make it easier to identify exactly which one is causing the trouble. Because rheumatoid conditions are usually very reactive, you will soon know whether you've eaten the wrong thing.

Along with the herbs mentioned above, anti-inflammatories like *Harpagophytum* (devil's claw), *Glycyrrhiza* (licorice) and *Dioscorea villosa* (wild yam) can be useful when treating rheumatoid arthritis. *Oenothera* (evening primrose oil) helps in about 70 percent of cases and combines well with fish oils to boost the body's production of anti-inflammatory hormones. *Urtica* (nettle) is a valuable system cleanser, too, while liver tonics like *Rumex crispus* (curled dock) and *Taraxacum officinale radix* (dandelion root) can help to calm down the auto-immune response. Although it takes persistence and frequent adjustments as the body gets used to whatever you are using and the inflammation flares up again, do not despair: there will always be something else to try.

Dandelions are a good liver tonic.

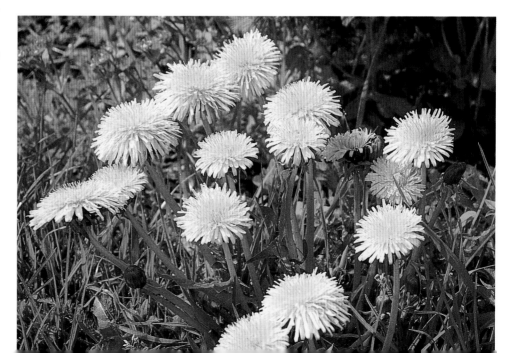

IMPROVING THE NERVOUS SYSTEM

The nervous system can always do with some help if you're not well. It's a vicious circle: stress can cause pain and other symptoms, certainly making them feel worse, while the symptoms themselves are a cause of stress. Sometimes a cup of *Matricaria* (chamomile) tea is all that you need to exit the spiral, but sometimes you'll need something stronger.

What doesn't help, in the long-term, is to turn to stimulants to get you through it. Many of our favorite, drinks – including tea and coffee – are herbal stimulants of one sort or another, which mostly rely on caffeine for their effect. Although they're fine when drunk in moderation, their overuse drains your nervous resources, making you feel worse. A better long-term strategy is to feed your nervous

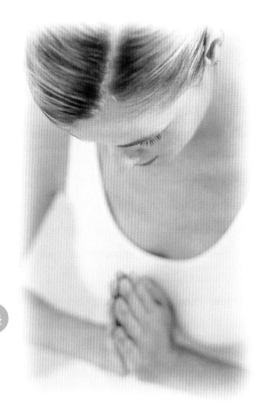

Yoga and meditation help you cope with stress.

74

system rather than depleting it. We all need to develop skills to enable us to cope with stress. If stimulants and drugs like alcohol and tobacco don't help – they may actually make things worse – then it's back to the usual list: exercise, a good diet, deep breathing and meditation, along with a good network of friends and a strong sense of self-worth. Yet we often need something more from time to time, so what do herbs have to offer?

Some herbs, like *Glycyrrhiza glabra* (licorice) and *Borago officinalis* (borage), support the adrenal

glands, while others, such as *Verbena* (vervain) and *Avena sativa* (oat straw), feed the nervous system. Still others work in a more obviously symptom-alleviating way, perhaps reducing anxiety or helping you slip into sleep, such as *Tilia* (lime flower), *Valeriana* (valerian) or *Matricaria* (chamomile). You can both combine them to suit your own needs and use most of them for as long as you like. The only herbs that should not be taken for too long are the ginsengs, *Panax ginseng* (Korean ginseng) and its cousins, and *Eleutherococcus senticosus* (Siberian ginseng), which, although they will pick you up and run with you, are too stimulating to take for more than about six weeks.

Some herbs will affect your mood more than others, while some will change your level of nervous arousal. Those that work well for depression include *Hypericum* (St. John's Wort), *Rosmarinus officinalis* (rosemary), *Borago officinalis* (borage) and *Tilia* (lime flower). A word of caution, though: reactive depression usually responds well to herbs, but clinical depression may require stronger measures. I've seen patients who have struggled for years with crippling depression while refusing to take orthodox drugs, although these can sometimes really make it possible to

ease back into normal life again. Remember, you haven't failed if you resort to such drugs – feeling bad about it will only makes matters worse – you can still use natural remedies to back up your drug therapy. When the time comes to give up the drugs, herbs will be there to help you. Likewise, manic depression and schizophrenia need more help than herbs can give, and knowing your limits is part of being effective.

I often see children who have been diagnosed as being hyperactive or suffering from attention-deficit disorder. This is an area in which you can usually do something without resorting to drugs. Because there are often food sensitivities at work, avoiding overloading their bodies with sugar and carbohydrates, additives and

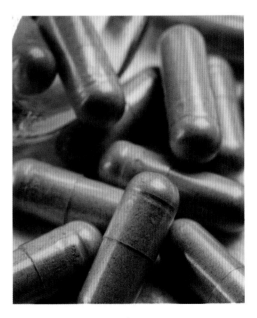

Ginseng: a temporary pick-me-up.

residues, along with the common troublemakers – wheat and dairy products – may make a big difference to children's behavior. Children can be surprisingly keen to give up the foods or drinks that they've been bingeing on once they realize how much better they feel without them. Some cranio-sacral work or hypnotherapy may help, too, particularly when the irritant foods have been removed from the child's diet. In the herbal department, strong relaxants like *Verbena* (vervain), and *Humulus* *lupulus* (hop) can help, combined with a gentle bitter, like *Taraxacum* (dandelion), and cleansing herbs like *Urtica* (nettle), *Trifolium pratense* (red clover), or *Galium aparine* (cleavers or goosegrass).

Insomnia is another form of nervous over-arousal, and there are a number of calming herbs, ranging from mild relaxants like *Matricaria* (German chamomile), which is ideal for young children, to more strongly sedative remedies like *Lactuca virosa* (wild lettuce). However, because

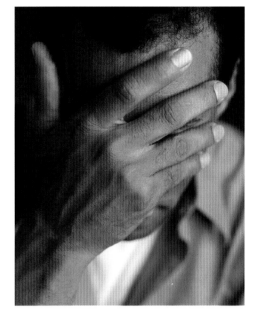

Depression: herbs can support the nervous system.

75

herbs are nowhere near as strong as many of the drugs that are available, people who have been used to relying on sleeping pills will not find it easy to make the transfer. What can often help is to take nervous-system remedies during the day, as well as a sleep-inducing remedy at bedtime. As your nervous system gets stronger, your sleeping problems should improve.

Problems that I see a great deal of are migraine and cluster headaches. And although sufferers may already have worked out for themselves what triggers their symptoms – perhaps a type of food – the underlying pattern

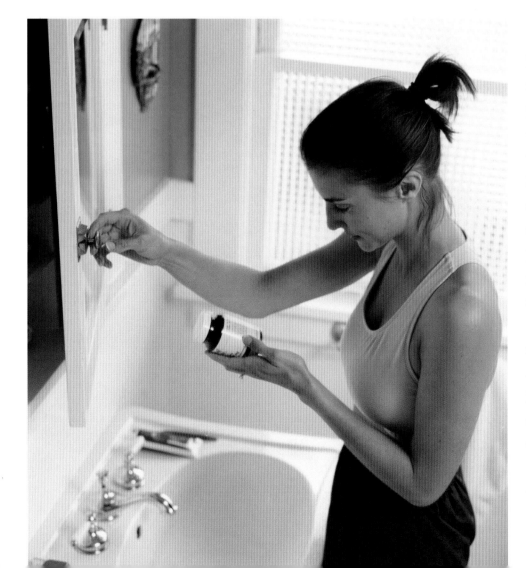

Watch out for additives.

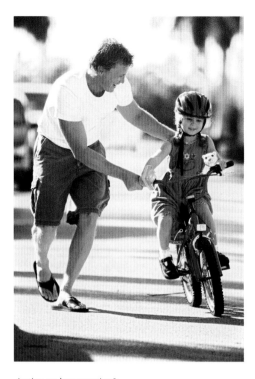

Active or hyperactive?

still remains. Migraine is a cyclical disorder: after an attack, you can't usually eat or do anything you want, but as you are building up toward another bout, your system becomes more and more sensitive, until the smallest thing sets off an attack. Again, the key to treating migraine and cluster headaches is to feed the nervous system. You may have heard of, or tried, *Tanacetum parthenium* (feverfew), which works by dilating the blood vessels in the neck and head that become constricted during some types of migraine attack. Although it

Head massage: touch is one of the most ancient healers.

can help a good deal, it doesn't address the problem at the deeper level. Because migraine is a visceral ailment – a cry for help from an over-taxed or depleted system – it responds gratefully to liver tonics and restoratives, as well as to symptom-focused remedies. Using *Verbena* (vervain), *Rosmarinus officinalis* (rosemary) and *Stachys betonica* (wood betony) will therefore serve you far better in the longer term.

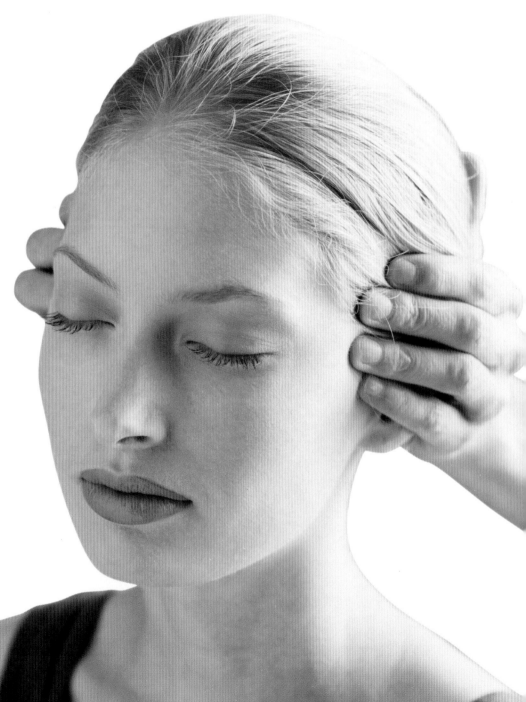

Urinary tract problems

There is a lot that herbs can do to improve the state of the tissues within the urinary tract, which may cause such problems as repeated infections, irritability and stress incontinence. For any infection more serious than cystitis, however, see a doctor: kidney problems need clearing up promptly, and may also require investigation.

For cystitis, the folk wisdom is to drink fruit or vegetable juice - particularly cranberry. Because this helps to make the urine alkaline, which makes bugs unhappy, this is sound advice. Cranberry will also assists anti-infective herbs, including *Thymus* (thyme), *Echinacea* (coneflower), and *Agropyron* (couch grass), to work. *Zea* (corn silk) helps to soothe any soreness and irritation.

Stress incontinence can be a problem in both women who have given birth and elderly people who have lost muscle tone. Infection may be at work, too, while anxiety can also play a part. Pelvic-floor exercises will help enormously – and remember that it is never too late to start them – while astringent herbs like *Plantago lanceolata* (ribwort) or *Equisetum arvense* (horsetail) will help to tighten up the muscles.

Fruit or vegetable juices can help prevent cystitis.

THE REPRODUCTIVE SYSTEM

There are many herbs that either stimulate the body's production or hormones or help replace them. I will be looking at a few in detail, but it is worth knowing about some of the others. Besides *Panax ginseng* (Korean ginseng), for example, there are herbs such as *Turnera damiana* (turnera) and *Smilax ornata* (sarsaparilla), that stimulate the production of "male" hormones like testosterone. Because low testosterone levels in both men and women can be one of the factors involved in having a low sex drive, these herbs have a well-deserved reputation as aphrodisiacs. They can alleviate conditions like undescended testicles and benign prostatic hypertrophy, and are tonic for both sexes, as they also have the

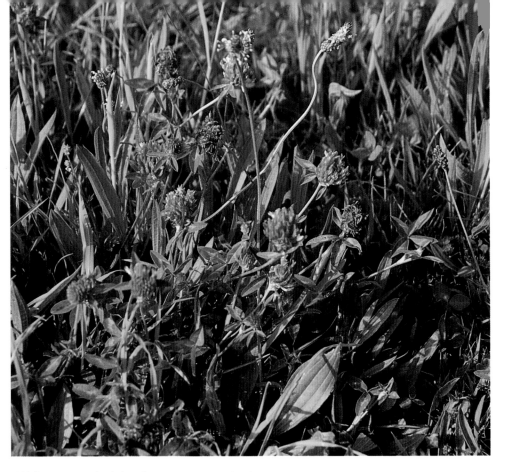

Trifolium pratense (red clover) supports estrogen levels.

power to boost low energy levels. (Caution: none of these herbs are suitable for pregnant or nursing women).

Apart from these herbs, there are few remedies that are specific to men (perhaps because there is less that can

go wrong within the male reproductive system). The main herbs that stimulate the "female" hormones include, for estrogen, *Angelica sinensis* (Chinese angelica or dong quai), *Salvia officinalis* (sage) and *Trifolium pratense* (red clover). For progesterone, there is *Vitex agnuscastus* (called chasteberry because medieval monks used it to depress their sex drive) and *Alchemilla vulgaris* (lady's mantle). A combination of these herbs can be useful to treat and normalize problems that could be due to a hormonal imbalance, including painful, irregular or heavy periods, premenstrual tension and menopausal symptoms.

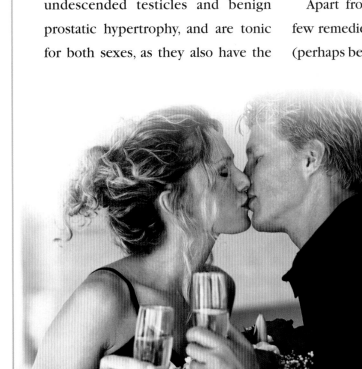

Herbs can boost your sex drive.

The herbs that specifically alleviate painful periods are *Viburnum opulus* (cramp bark), an anti-spasmodic, and herbs that are beneficial to the circulation, such as *Zingiber* (ginger) and *Rosmarinus officinalis* (rosemary). Very heavy periods can be treated with uterine tonics like *Rubus idaeus* (raspberry leaf) or *Alchemilla vulgaris* (lady's mantle), but I'd also advise you to see a doctor in case fibroids, endometriosis or some other problem is present that may need further treatment. *Oenothera* (evening primrose oil) is worth trying, to alleviate pre-menstrual tension, and can be taken together with *Vitex agnus-castus* (chasteberry) and nervous-system supporters like *Valeriana* (valerian). Because they work on the underlying imbalance rather than the monthly symptoms, it's best to take the herbs all of the time, and not just before your period.

Women who are going through menopause may either experience no problems at all or have a very rough ride. There is some evidence that an over-rich diet can make symptoms like hot flashes more likely, so reduc-

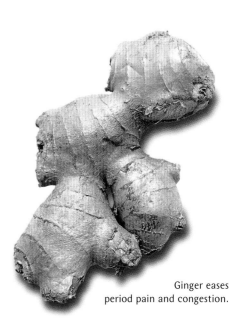

Ginger eases period pain and congestion.

ing your intake of sugar and fats, along with coffee, may be a useful step. Eating more estrogen-rich foods, particularly soya beans and other pulses, can help to replace estrogen. If you are one of the unlucky women who suffer from hot flashes, palpitations, mood swings and other symptoms of menopause, the first herbs for you to try are *Salvia* (sage), *Leonurus cardiaca* (motherwort) and *Hypericum* (St. John's Wort). Herbs that support the nervous-system such as *Avena sativa* (oat straw) and *Passiflora incarnata* (passionflower) will help too. When menopause starts, it is worth testing

Soybeans are rich in estrogen.

79

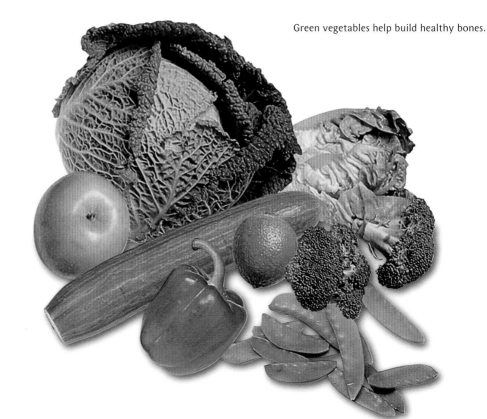

Green vegetables help build healthy bones.

to see if you are likely to be prone to osteoporosis. If so, make sure that you have plenty of calcium-rich foods, like dark-green vegetables and sesame seeds, herbs like *Equisetum arvense* (horsetail), and *Urtica* (nettle), and that you take regular, weight-bearing exercise. Despite these measures, your doctor may recommend hormone replacement therapy (HRT), which, although I do not recommend it lightly, can be a life-saver for some women. Herbs can also help to deal with any unwanted side effects of HRT, but consult a qualified practitioner rather than trying to treat yourself.

Most women will have an encounter with an infection of one sort or another, from vaginal thrush to the deep, anaerobic infections that

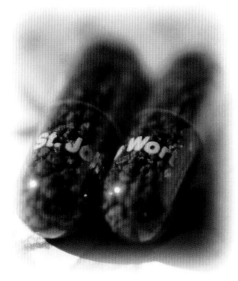

St. John's Wort can help you through menopause.

can lead to period pains and fertility problems. Although sexually transmitted diseases must be seen and treated by a doctor, two common types of infection are often treated by herbalists and other complementary therapists: persistent thrush and pelvic inflammatory disease (PID).

It is possible to treat thrush, but it can take months, or even years, before the affected tissues have recovered to the point where they are no longer vulnerable to new infection. Taking *Allium sativum* (garlic), *Calendula* (marigold) and *Thymus* (thyme) will slowly, but surely, change the situation for the better, because they tone and soothe the congested vaginal walls,

thereby making thrush – and other infections – very unwelcome. Dietary factors play a part, too, but, while anti-candida diets place a lot of emphasis on avoiding yeast-rich foods, I am not convinced that this makes any difference. I have seen people who have been faithfully following the "candida diet" (and a dull regime it is, too) for months, achieving nothing but a loss of well-being, who have begun to respond positively to herbal medicine within weeks. To bring relief when your vaginal tissues are sore and itching, a cream made with the oils of *Thymus vulgaris* (thyme) and *Melaleuca alternifolia* (tea tree) will prove a blessing.

80

Massage with
lavender oil to ease abdominal pain.

Pelvic inflammatory disease (PID) is often used as an umbrella diagnosis for vague pelvic pain that doesn't respond to treatment. The deep-seated infections of the womb, fallopian tubes and ovaries can not only be notoriously resistant to antibiotic treatment, but may survive at sub clinical levels that do not show up in tests. Inflammation can arise as a result of endometriosis or other disease processes, including infection, or it can be caused by adhesions following surgery. Whatever the cause of PID, its symptoms are many and varied, including painful periods, discharge or bleeding between periods, twinges or aching (sometimes felt as lower-back pain), mild fevers for no apparent reason, and chronically low energy. Sexual intercourse can be painful, and fertility may be lowered.

Pelvic problems can affect fertility.

81

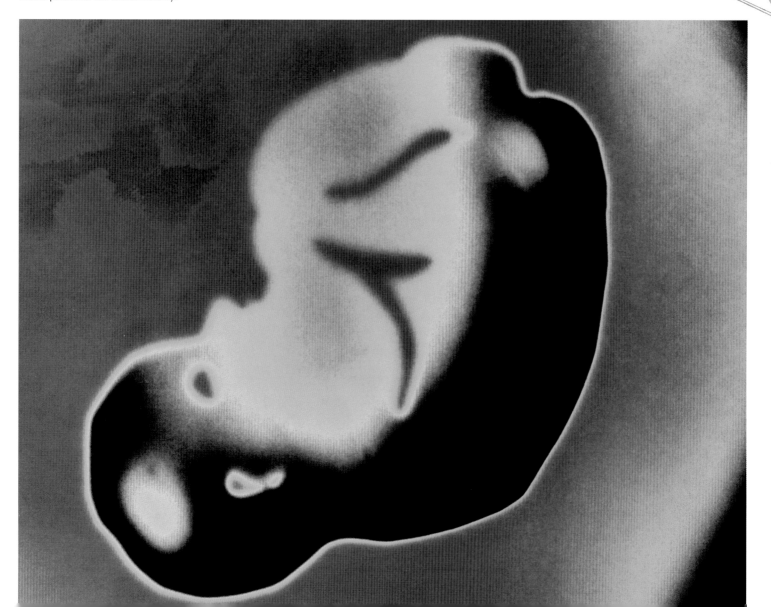

Running helps flush out the system.

Yoga can relieve
pelvic congestion.

bring relief, as can hydrotherapy (using hot and cold baths). Gentle exercise, of the kind that stretches, tones, and relieves pelvic congestion – for example, walking, swimming, yoga and even singing – is essential. The important thing is to find an exercise that you enjoy, rather than following a program because it is good for you. It is my strong belief that increasing the joy that you experience in life is crucial to shaking off PID, so finding things you like doing should be part of the prescription!

The herbal treatment for PID is much the same whatever its cause: circulatory herbs, such as *Zingiber* (ginger) and *Rosmarinus officinalis* (rosemary), and lots of anti-infectives and anti-inflammatories like *Echinacea* (coneflower), *Calendula* (marigold), *Thymus* (thyme), and *Allium sativum* (garlic). Gentle abdominal massage using the oils of *Lavandula vera* (lavender) and *Melissa officinalis* (lemon balm) can

Herbs can give you gentle support throughout your pregnancy.

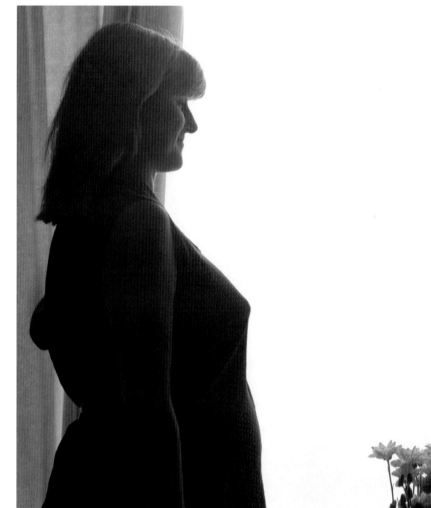

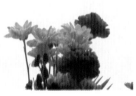

ed, the man's sperm count quadrupled during that time, and the couple went on to have two children – so it can be done!) Women may have damaged fallopian tubes or ovaries, problems that lie beyond the reach of herbal remedies, although, as we have seen, a lot can be done to improve circulation, reduce inflammation and rebalance hormones. Not only can tonic herbs be used alongside fertility drugs, they can also help to restore your natural cycle after you've stopped taking the drugs. The conception process can be very stressful, in which case relaxing herbs will be of help to both partners. (Never overestimate your ability to cope: use all of the support you can get and try to give yourselves time out occasionally.)

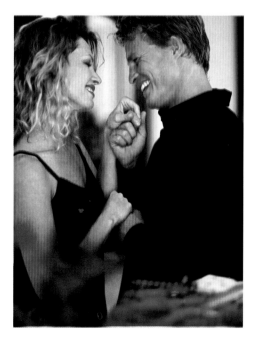

The first step on the way...

The last topic that I'll discuss in this section is pregnancy. If you are having difficulty conceiving or are experiencing problems during pregnancy or while nursing, you may want to try to treat them yourself. If you do not get the results that you are hoping for, however, see a qualified practitioner.

Having difficulty conceiving can, of course, stem from either of the prospective parents or from the inter-action between them. Both should check to see if they have any infections and, if so, treat them in whatever way works best. If the problem is a low sperm count, the testosterone-stimulating herbs listed on page 78 should prove useful, along with others. (Remember that because it takes three months to produce fresh sperm, you will not see positive results any earlier. In one case I treat-

When you become pregnant, you should ideally try to avoid any kind of medication, at least for the first three months. Having said that, you can safely use herb teas like *Matricaria* (chamomile), *Mentha piperita* (peppermint) or *Zingiber* (ginger) for morning sickness and indigestion (see a herbal practitioner if this is not enough), while Urtica (nettle) will boost your iron levels. If you have reason to fear a miscarriage, you could take *Viburnum opulus* (cramp bark) with *Valeriana* (valerian) to help you to relax; if there is any sign of bleeding, go to bed immediately.

During the last two or three months of pregnancy, you could take *Rubus idaeus* (raspberry leaf) to prepare your womb for labor. If things are not progressing well during labor itself, try *Caulophyllum thalictroides* (blue cohosh) to get the process moving along. If, on the other hand, the contractions are fast and furious and you are feeling out of control, try *Cimicifuga racemosa* (black cohosh) and *Viburnum opulus* (cramp bark) to take the edge off the pain and enable you to center yourself.

After the birth of your baby, *Rubus idaeus* (raspberry leaf) and *Caulophyllum thalictroides* (blue cohosh) will encourage your womb to return to normal. Many herbs traditionally stimulate milk production, such as

Urtica (nettle), *Carum carvi* (caraway) and *Foeniculum vulgare* (fennel), but if you are trying to reduce your milk supply, *Salvia officinalis* (sage) will help. For mastitis and breast abscesses, try *Echinacea* (cone-

flower), *Taraxacum officinale radix* (dandelion root), *Galium aparine* (cleavers or goosegrass), and *Viola odorata* (sweet violet), which can be taken internally and applied externally as a lotion, cream or compress.

Nettle boosts iron levels and aids milk production.

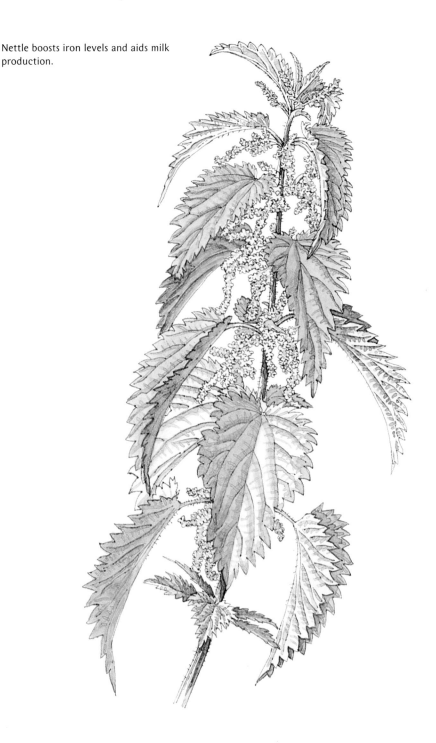

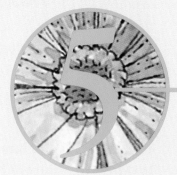

Herb directory

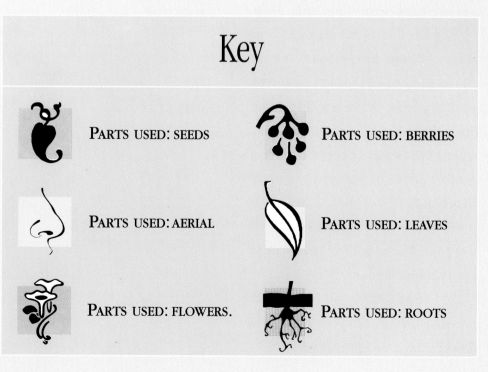

Key

PARTS USED: SEEDS		PARTS USED: BERRIES	
PARTS USED: AERIAL		PARTS USED: LEAVES	
PARTS USED: FLOWERS.		PARTS USED: ROOTS	

Achillea millefolium (yarrow)

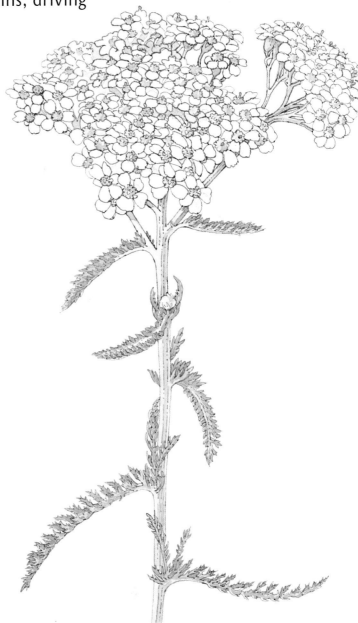

Achillea is a herb with backbone, so if you need to stiffen your resolve or prepare for a challenge, think Achillea. It is named after the Greek warrior hero Achilles, who was invulnerable except for his Achilles' heel, and it is a good friend to warriors of either sex. Achillea helps to boost your vitality before battle and to heal any wounds afterward, whether it's the old-fashioned sort of fight or a more complicated, modern kind of conflict. It does this mainly by stimulating the circulation, flushing slow-moving blood from the veins, driving blood into the capillaries, readying the limbs for action and speeding up healing. Achillea can even make you sweat, which aids the fever process when you have an acute infection, and it is one of the most useful herbs for lowering blood pressure, too.

The virtues of Achillea do not end there, however, because it contains oils that are anti-inflammatory, antiseptic, and refreshing to the spirit (in Sweden, it is traditionally added to beer to banish melancholy). The oil also soothes muscle spasms and heads off the allergic reactions that cause the symptoms of asthma and hay fever; for some people, sniffing Achillea oil can be enough to ward off an attack.

For fever, Achillea combines well with *Sambucus* (elder) and *Mentha piperita* (peppermint).

To bring down high blood pressure, use Achillea with *Tilia* (lime flower) and *Crataegus* (hawthorn).

Agropyron repens (couch grass)

Did you think that couch grass (*Agropyron repens*) was just a gardener's nightmare? If so, think again, because it has a secret gift to offer: the creeping roots that gardeners try so hard to get rid of are a powerful remedy for all forms of irritation and inflammation within the urinary tract. Cystitis, urethritis, prostatitis and benign prostatic hypertrophy – all respond well to Agropyron. You can use it as a "background" remedy for kidney stones as well, although these may need further treatment.

As well as soothing inflammation, Agropyron has slightly anti-infective properties, but in cases of infection its effectiveness will be much enhanced if you use it with *Thymus* (thyme), *Echinacea* (coneflower), *Barosma betulina* (buchu) or *Arctostaphylos uva-ursi* (bearberry).

For prostatic enlargement, use it with *Smilax ornata* (sarsaparilla), *Turnera diffusa* (turnera) or *Serenoa repens* (sabal).

87

Allium sativum (garlic)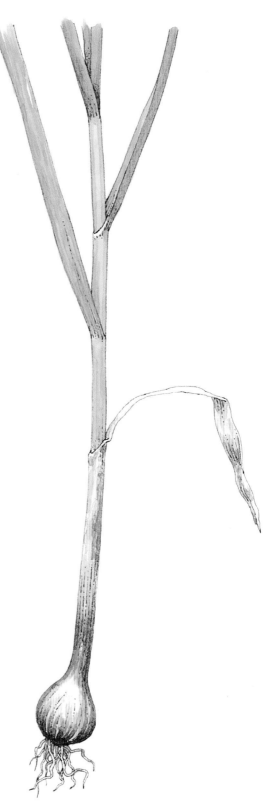

It is the cloves, or corms, of *Allium sativum* that we use, both in cooking and in healing. When added to food, its action gives us a clue about its first medicinal use: besides enhancing the flavor of many dishes, it also helps us to digest them. By adding its fire to food, it warms up the digestive system, stimulating the digestive juices to flow and improving the absorption of nutrients.

It also discourages parasites and other unhelpful potential inhabitants from setting up home in the gut, which leads us on to its second main use: *Allium sativum* is a wonderful anti-infective herb that discourages or eliminates all sorts of infective agents, from parasites to bacteria, fungi and viruses. Before the discovery of antibiotics, *Allium sativum* was routinely used to combat infection, and even if you are on a course of antibiotics, taking it can still be useful because of its beneficial action on the gut and helpful gut flora. Its anti-infective property is mainly due to its powerful essential oil, which diffuses easily into the tissues of the body. (I am told, although I have never checked this out for myself, that if you eat raw garlic, you can detect it – by the smell, of course – in the soles of your feet twenty minutes later!)

Allium sativum is therefore effective against infection anywhere in the body, from vaginal thrush to athlete's foot to lung and throat problems. It is particularly useful for treating chest infections because it also loosens and promotes the flow of mucus within the lungs, cleansing them from the base upward. In addition, secreting *Allium sativum* in your sweat makes you a less than appetizing target for mosquitoes and other creatures that attack the skin – it's a bit like having a personal force field around you. The only disadvantage is that people tend to be repelled by the smell if you overdo it! And a word of caution here: because the oil that does the magic is also the source of the smell, if you take any preparations of *Allium sativum* that have been deodorized or processed in any way to remove the smell, they will not be very effective against infection. The best way to take Allium sativum is, therefore, to chop up the raw cloves and swallow them with water. Failing that, buy capsules containing the pure oil, with nothing added or removed.

The third gift that *Allium sativum* has to offer is its effect on circulation: it promotes blood flow, lowers blood cholesterol, helps to combat – and maybe even reverse – hardening of the arteries and reduces stickiness of the blood. This makes it invaluable for treating cases of high blood pressure or cholesterol, and for thinning the blood following a stroke or a heart attack, for example – three standard-sized garlic-oil capsules are the equivalent of one small aspirin in this regard. Be careful, however: if you are already taking warfarin or another medication to thin your blood, consult your doctor before taking *Allium sativum*, because it may upset the balance.

A standard dose of *Allium sativum* is one hazelnut-sized clove, chopped up and swallowed raw, or three standard-sized garlic-oil capsules. If you succumb to an acute infection, however, you can safely flood your system with *Allium sativum* – indeed, the more you take, the better. Although nine to twelve capsules will do the trick for most people, your body will let you know its own limit by producing loose stools.

If I had to choose just a handful of herbs to work with, *Allium sativum* would be one of them. Its potent drying and fire-raising qualities would be hard to replace: in congested chest conditions like chronic bronchitis or

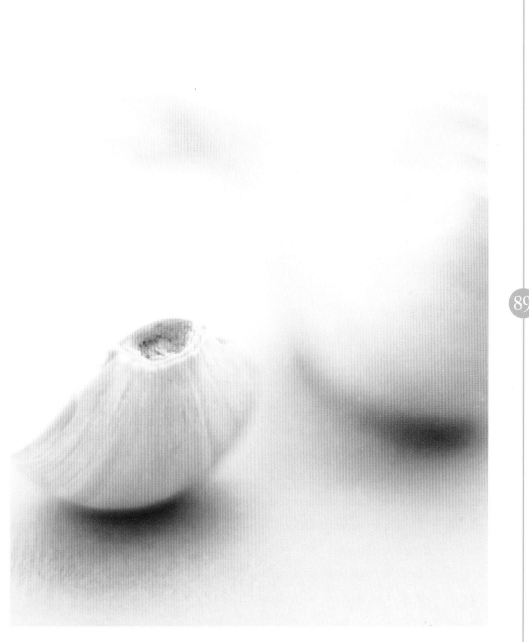

Garlic: a potent fire raiser.

asthma, for example, introducing garlic is like kindling a bonfire in the middle of a swamp. Occasionally you will come across someone who is already too "hot" for *Allium sativum* (they will usually already know this because they find it hard to digest),

who will respond better to gentler digestive herbs like *Thymus vulgaris* (thyme) or *Matricaria* (chamomile). In general, however, *Allium sativum* should be in everyone's herbal medicine chest.

Aloe vera (aloe)

Aloe vera and its Aloe cousins are highly prized for the juice in their leaves, which is a potent anti-inflammatory that takes the sting out of sunburn, burns and sores of all types. Keep a plant on the kitchen windowsill, and it will reward you with a vigorous supply of succulent leaves, each filled to bursting point with healing gel; you can break one off when you need it and apply the juice directly to the skin. Rarely does the herb world offer us a gift so straightforward and also so generous.

Taking *Aloe vera* internally is less straightforward, however. The juice contains a substance called aloe-emodin, a powerful purgative, which, if you take it in its raw state, has effects that are certainly not healing. Before *Aloe vera* can be taken internally, it must, therefore, be processed to remove all trace of aloe-emodin. (Strictly speaking, the many preparations of *Aloe vera* that are on the market for internal use are thus not whole herbal remedies.) Once its fangs have been removed, however, *Aloe vera* becomes such a valuable remedy that it has gained a secure place in the herbal pharmacopoeia.

The claims made for *Aloe vera* preparations are legendary, causing it to have become touted as yet another cure-all. Although its anti-inflammatory properties are both very impressive and helpful for treating many conditions in which inflammation features, if I had to pick only one application for *Aloe vera*, it would be for treating bowel problems, from irritable bowel through ulcerative colitis to diverticular disease. Together with diet management, *Aloe vera* is a faithful ally in this respect, and it combines happily with other herbs, such as *Melissa* (lemon balm), *Symphytum* (comfrey) and *Matricaria* (chamomile), too.

Calendula officinalis (marigold)

It is the petals or whole flower heads of *Calendula officinalis* that are used in herbal medicine and, as the seventeenth-century English herbalist Nicholas Culpeper said, just looking at them is enough to draw the "evil humors" out of you. Indeed, their bright, optimistic, golden color gives a clue to their healing properties: cleansing, toning and stimulating. Calendula is both astringent, helping to close up wounds and tone the skin, and anti-infective, discouraging bacteria, fungal and viral infections from taking hold. It is also an anti-inflammatory, taking the heat out of throbbing wounds or "hot" skin conditions like nettle rash. Calendula cream, which can be applied to cuts and abrasions, sunburn and insect bites, is an essential ingredient in any first aid kit.

Calendula's qualities also make it superb for treating longer-term skin problems like acne, athlete's foot and thrush, which it will gently, but persistently, discourage until they give up and disappear. Internally, too, it is the first herb of choice to treat all of the manifestations of candida, from bloating and gas to vaginal thrush. It helps to re-establish healthy gut flora when the bacterial balance has been disrupted, for example, by illness or antibiotics. Working higher up, in the stomach and small intestine, it will heal inflammation and stomach ulcers.

By taking the inflammation from emotional states, helping a person to draw their energies together and cope with crises and traumas, Calendula brings light to dark places in the mind, too. Calendula combines well with *Symphytum* (comfrey) as a cream or lotion for external wounds, and with *Thymus vulgaris* (thyme), internally and externally, for thrush.

91

Crataegus oxyacanthoides (hawthorn)

Crataegus is a restorative food for the heart whose unique combination of ingredients tones the blood vessels and also improves the efficiency of the heart's action. If you have high blood pressure, Crataegus will work to bring it down, while if your blood pressure is lower than it should be (enough to make you feel faint and dizzy at times), it will tend to rise as the heart becomes stronger. Crataegus can, therefore, also help when there are irregularities in the heartbeat (arrhythmias), angina and swollen ankles due to heart problems. Crataegus can be safely used in the long-term to lend solid support to anyone who is suffering from these problems or who has even developed heart failure or had a heart attack. And, if taken continuously, it will help to prevent hardening of the arteries and may even play a part in its reversal.

Research has shown that if a careful program of heart care is followed, it is not only possible to recover completely from a heart attack, but to reach a higher level of fitness than before. Such a program could include regular exercise (a moderate amount at first and then building gradually), a diet that is rich in fruit and vegetables and low in saturated fats, and the daily use of Crataegus and other supportive herbs. It could also include learning stress-management skills, and taking a long, hard look at the lifestyle that has given rise to such a life-threatening crisis.

For high blood pressure, Crataegus works well with *Achillea* (yarrow) and *Tilia* (lime flower).

92

Echinacea spp. (coneflower)

Several varieties of Echinacea have medicinal value, including *E. angustifolia*, *purpurea* and *pallida*, of which *E. angustifolia* is generally held to be the most useful. All varieties of Echinacea are, however, powerful, no-nonsense allies in our efforts to become, and stay, well. Not only do they directly inhibit the growth of bacteria, but – much more importantly – they support our immune systems, thereby helping us to help ourselves.

People often regard Echinacea as a sort of herbal antibiotic, but this misses the point entirely. Antibiotics may rid us of "hostile" bacteria, but they also kill the "friendly" bacteria within the gut, are a burden for the liver to break down and do nothing to clear up the debris of infection or to restore the tissues to health. Echinacea, on the other hand, is what the old herbalists used to call a "blood-cleanser": it stimulates the circulation and flushes out, and encourages, the elimination of waste products. It acts much like a slightly bullying nurse who sweeps away the sickroom clutter and flings open the windows, to aid and encourage a swift convalescence.

There is no substance, at least in my experience, to the idea that you should only take Echinacea in short bursts to prevent it from losing its beneficial effect. On the contrary, I

93

acute illness, you can raise the dose to as much as 5ml of Echinacea tincture (since Echinacea does not taste good, a tincture is better than a tea), taken every two hours or so. Over the long-term, taking a few drops a day may be enough to keep your immune system on the alert.

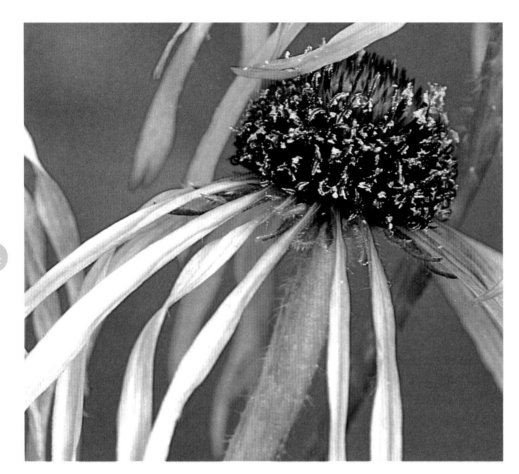

Echinacea angustifolia (coneflower) is a powerful aid to boosting the immunity.

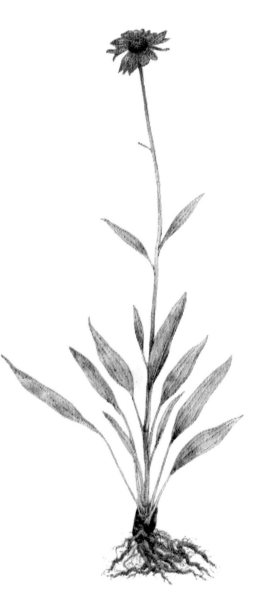

believe that it is a herb that can safely be taken over a prolonged period of time to give long-term protection and improve the immune-system efficiency of people who have been prone to infections. It can, however, sometimes prove too powerful for people who have become very debilitated, particularly if they are suffering from post-viral fatigue syndrome or have very poor circulation, in which case gentler, slower methods of treatment

– persuasion rather than pushing – are needed.

Echinacea performs well when combined with *Achillea* (yarrow), for example, to boost the circulation and help to raise the body temperature in cases of acute infection, or with *Glycyrrhiza glabra* (licorice) in working to clear the chest, soothe the stomach or quell inflammation, depending on what type of infection you are trying to treat. In instances of

Filipendula ulmaria (meadowsweet)

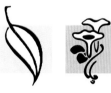

Filipendula ulmaria's waterside habitat is a clue to its action: gently warming, but not drying like so many of the "hot" herbs whose natural home is the dry, stony hills of the Mediterranean, such as *Thymus* (thyme), *Salvia* (sage) and *Rosmarinus* (rosemary). Its effect on the spirit is softening, warming and expansive, helping to dissolve any "stuck" feelings and rigid thought patterns. In the words of the old herbalists, *Filipendula ulmaria* "makes the heart merrie."

Its action is similar on the physical level, making it particularly effective in two main areas. The first is in the relief of rheumatic problems: pain, swelling and stiffness in the muscles and joints respond well to Filipendula. Among its useful ingredients is a significant amount of salicylic acid, which is the active ingredient in aspirin, and Filipendula can therefore do anything that aspirin can, although the salicylic acid that it contains is less concentrated than within aspirin. This is an advantage, not a drawback, because included among its other ingredients are compounds that help to buffer the undesirable effects of salicylic acid. (If you have taken aspirin, or any of its fellow non-steroidal, anti-inflammatory drugs (NSAIDS), you may know that they can irritate the stomach lining to the extent of causing gastric erosions when over-used.) Filipendula, on the other hand, actually encourages the healing of gastric erosions and ulcers (its second main use in medical herbalism) by reducing the amount of acid in the stomach and soothing inflammation.

Use it for any signs of stomach trouble, from heartburn (reflux esophagitis), indigestion and peptic ulcers to mild diarrhea. It is also excellent for treating stomach upsets in children.

Ginkgo biloba (ginkgo)

Although it is less powerful than some of the other circulatory herbal stimulants I have mentioned, *Ginkgo biloba* has a gentle and persistent action, making it the ideal support for anyone who has either had a stroke or has reason to fear one. It works by effecting a gradual improvement in circulation, and the health of the blood vessels.

Because its effectiveness will not fade away over time, you can take Ginkgo for as long as you like. (In fact, for conditions like tinnitus, you will need to give it as much as six months before you can ascertain how much it is helping.) Likewise, for long-term problems like chronic migraines or forgetfulness, it will provide unobtrusive, but substantial, back-up.

For stroke management and prevention, try taking it with *Allium sativum* (garlic) and *Crataegus* (hawthorn). For tinnitus, combine it with *Hypericum* (St. John's Wort). *Rosmarinus officinalis* (rosemary) is a good companion to Ginkgo when treating absent-mindedness and forgetfulness.

96

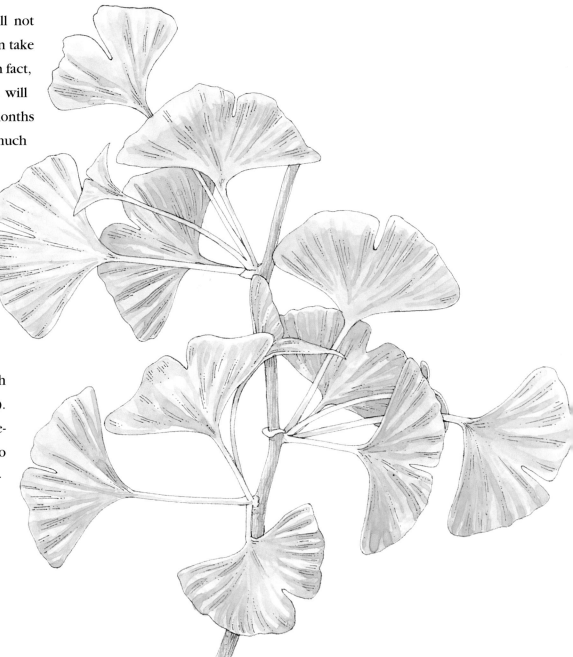

Glycyrrhiza glabra (licorice)

Glycyrrhiza glabra is one of the herbal heavyweights. It has a number of actions that together add up to a potent healing remedy for peptic ulcers (and before the advent of drugs like Zantac, *Glycyrrhiza glabra* was the doctors' first choice). If you chew an old-fashioned licorice stick, it will coat the stomach lining with a thick, protective layer that is soothing, anti-spasmodic and anti-inflammatory. At the same time, underlying the sweet taste that has earned it a place in candy stores is a bitterness that cools the stomach and encourages digestive juices (other than stomach acid) to flow, with the result that it benefits the whole of the digestive system. It also works on the respiratory system, encouraging the production of mucus and helping to resolve bronchitis, making it a useful ingredient in any cough remedy.

The main reason why it plays a part in so many herbal prescriptions, however, is that it supports the action of the adrenal glands. *Glycyrrhiza glabra* contains plant steroids that both support the adrenals in the production of steroid hormones and can heighten, or replace, them if the adrenals are not producing enough. These steroids are the body's main method of dealing with inflammation of all sorts, which means that you can use *Glycyrrhiza glabra* to treat any inflammatory problem, from arthritis to eczema. And if the adrenal glands need a bit of help after coping with stress - physical or emotional - *Glycyrrhiza glabra* will act as their staunch supporter.

In traditional Chinese medicine, *Glycyrrhiza uralensis* (a first cousin to *G. glabra*) appears in around 90 percent of all prescriptions. This is because it is said to open the channels for all of the other herbs to do their work, and when you consider what its actions are, this explanation makes a lot of sense. The only time when it would be better to leave it out of a prescription is if you are suffering from hypertension because it has occasionally been shown to push high blood pressure up even further.

Glycyrrhiza glabra combines well with *Filipendula* (meadowsweet) and *Symphytum* (comfrey) for treating stomach ulcers. For alleviating sore throats and bronchitis, it works well with *Thymus* (thyme) and *Echinacea* (coneflower). Try it with *Verbena* (vervain) for adrenal support.

Hypericum perforatum (St. John's Wort)

Hypericum perforatum is a gentle herb that helps to ease you through transitions of any kind. Its yellow flowers appear at midsummer, and taking it bestows some of that summer light upon you, enabling you to see your way through troubled times. Because it doesn't make its presence felt immediately – you'll be taking it for about six weeks before you start to feel the benefit – if you're using it as part of a drug-withdrawal program, start taking it well before you begin to reduce the drug dosage.

Hypericum perforatum outsells Prozac in Germany, and has done so for some years. It is excellent for alleviating mild depression, tranquilizing without sedating and lifting your mood without suppressing your feelings or creating a dependency situation. For anyone who is in emotional pain, *Hypericum perforatum* will be a friend in need.

It helps nervous-system problems on the physical level, too, gently easing the pain of neuralgia (you can use it externally as well) and shingles, for example. Indeed, wherever there is damage to the nerves, Hypericum perforatum may be of help.

The third main use for *Hypericum perforatum* is during menopause, when it helps to dampen down hot flashes and excessive sweating.

For treating depression, it combines well with *Verbena* (vervain), *Avena sativa* (oat straw), *Scutellaria laterifolia* (skullcap) or *Piper methysticum* (kava).

For neuralgia, try it with *Achillea* (yarrow), *Lactuca virosa* (wild lettuce) and a little *Capsicum minimum* (cayenne).

For menopausal problems, combine it with *Salvia* (sage) and *Leonurus* (motherwort).

(Caution: there are some reservations to be aware of regarding *Hypericum perforatum*. First, it has long been known to cause photosensitive reactions in some people. Second, and more recently, it has been shown to affect the uptake of some orthodox drugs, including warfarin and digoxin, cyclosporin, oral contraceptives and some anti-depressants that act on the central nervous system. If you are already on any medication, the golden rule is to check with a doctor or herbalist before taking *Hypericum perforatum* and to have your blood regularly monitored to ensure that the drugs' correct levels are being maintained.)

Matricaria recutita (chamomile)

Matricaria recutita used to be known as "the plants' physician" because when it was grown near plants that were not thriving, their health tended to improve. In the same way, if you include it in a mixture of herbs, it can often enhance the preparation's effectiveness by improving digestion so that the herbs can be better absorbed, gently boosting the circulation and smoothing away tension, too. Although it is more of a nurse than a physician, it is the best sort of nurse: gentle but firm, taking the patient in hand and restoring heart and hope.

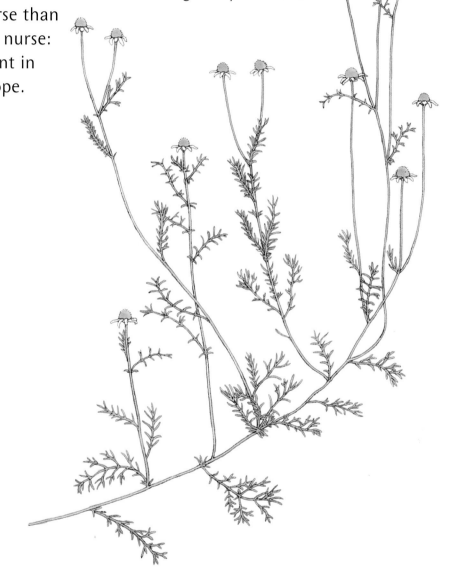

For all of these reasons, *Matricaria recutita* is a remedy par excellence for children. Many children's ailments involve stomach ache, and *Matricaria recutita* is in its element here because it soothes spasms and gently encourages the flow of digestive juices. It also works on the anxiety that so often goes with being ill when you are a child. A cup of chamomile tea at bedtime will help an excited child to slip into sleep.

Don't assume that because a remedy is good for children it will not be strong enough for adults – *Matricaria recutita* will work just as well for grown-ups as for children. Some people hate the taste of it, however, so check that he or she will drink it before making a calming mixture for someone. Taken regularly, this herb is capable of helping to heal an inflamed stomach or an irritable bowel, or of taking the edge off feelings of fear and nervousness. Made into a cream or a wash, it will also soothe the irritation of sunburn or eczema.

99

Melissa officinalis (lemon balm)

Melissa officinalis is one of the many herbs that we particularly value for their fragrant volatile oils, but volatile oils, as their name implies, are fragile and easily lost. That of *Melissa officinalis* is especially elusive, and most commercially dried samples do not have much of its smell left. If you dry some carefully yourself, however, you will be amazed by the intensity of both its smell and flavor. And, because it is the oil that works much of the magic, you'll also be rewarded with a far more powerful remedy.

*M*elissa officinalis has a particular talent for treating abdominal problems and works on the gut and uterus alike to soothe cramps and relax tension. It is excellent for gently calming and toning an irritable bowel, thereby encouraging the bowel's natural processes to flow smoothly again. It also eases period pains and can help to alleviate hot flashes.

Like most volatile-oil-rich herbs, *Melissa officinalis* helps to lift feelings of anxiety and depression (in the words of Culpeper, it "driveth away troublesome cares . . . arising from melancholy or black choler"). Its action is protective and gently enclosing, making it a good remedy for people who need to be held together as the wounds caused by a physical or emotional trauma heal.

For treating an irritable bowel, an excellent herbal combination is Melissa, *Symphytum* (comfrey) and *Mentha piperita* (peppermint). This has an immediate first-aid effect that eases the pain of gas and stomach cramps. You could also try massaging a few drops of Melissa oil into the stomach if it is sore. In the longer term, drinking this tea regularly will slowly re-educate the bowel, enabling it to relax and "unlearn" any bad habits.

Mentha piperita (peppermint)

Although many varieties of *Mentha* (mint) can be used in herbal medicine, *Mentha piperita* is the best remedy for the ailments that we will be looking at. Its oil is intensely aromatic, with an underlying bitterness that adds to its pungency. Unlike most of the volatile oils that we value in cooking, as well as healing, it is unusual in that it has a cooling, rather than a warming, effect. In medicinal terms, this means that it can provide a useful counterpoint to the "hotter" herbs. It also means that it should not be over-used, however.

Mentha piperita combines well with *Sambucus nigra* (elder) and *Achillea millefolium* (yarrow), for example, to make an effective tea for the relief of colds, flu and chest infections. To treat sinusitis, you could make an inhalation preparation with the essential oils of *Mentha piperita*, *Eucalyptus globulus* (eucalyptus), *Pinus sylvestris* (pine) and *Thymus vulgaris* (thyme). Add a couple of drops of each to a bowl of near-boiling water before breathing in the steam, gently at first, until it penetrates the blocked sinuses. (If you do not have their oils, strong infusions of any of those herbs will do.) Note that using *Mentha piperita* on its own would have too much of a cooling and drying effect, making it more of an irritant than an aid.

Similarly, to treat digestive troubles, *Mentha piperita* works best in combination with other herbs. With the power to dispel gas, ease stomach pains and colic and lift nausea instantly, it also discourages intestinal parasites, although it will not get rid of them completely. Although tea made of this herb alone can be a wonderfully refreshing remedy for indigestion, too much of it may actually bring on nausea rather than relieve it. It's therefore much more effective to mix it with herbs like *Matricaria* (chamomile), *Melissa* (lemon balm) or *Tilia* (lime flower).

(Caution: the essential oil is not suitable for babies.)

Oenothera biennis (evening primrose)

The oil extracted from the seeds of *Oenothera biennis* has one great quality: it contains a relatively large amount of gamma-linolenic acid (GLA), which is present in other seeds, too, but in smaller quantities. This substance is one of the precursors of a prostaglandin hormone which we make within our bodies and which calms down inflammation. Although we can normally synthesize GLA as well, there are certain conditions that stop our bodies from doing this, including obesity, stress and diabetes. When this happens, we slowly run out of our supply of GLA and are thus more vulnerable to the effects of inflammation. Enter *Oenothera biennis*, closely followed by a few other rich sources of GLA, notably *Borago officinalis* (borage or starflower) and *Rubus nigra* (blackcurrant) seeds.

A great deal of research has been done on *Oenothera biennis*, and we now understand rather well what it can, and cannot, do. Its uses are many. When used to treat multiple sclerosis, for instance, it can both lengthen the time between attacks and make them milder. It helps 70 percent of the people who suffer from rheumatoid arthritis and almost the same percentage of eczema-sufferers, too. In addition, it is effective in alleviating premenstrual tension and the symptoms of menopause.

When addressing all of these conditions, you will need to take a fairly high dose of *Oenothera biennis* for three months before the deficit of GLA within the body is made up (many people who have found it ineffective have just not been taking enough). During this period, the dose for an adult with rheumatoid arthritis or eczema is eight 500mg capsules daily, while for those with premenstrual tension or menopause it is six. At the end of three months, you can reduce the dose to a maintenance level of one or two 500mg capsules daily or perhaps stop taking it altogether. *Oenothera biennis* is relatively expensive but given its impressive track record, it is worth persisting with.

When treating rheumatoid arthritis, you could also use other anti-inflammatories, such as *Glycyrrhiza* (licorice) or *Dioscorea* (wild yam), together with *Achillea* (yarrow), which gives circulatory support.

For eczema, try it with blood-cleansers like *Urtica* (nettle) and *Rumex crispus* (curled dock), a liver tonic, such as *Verbena* (vervain), and soothing herbs like *Matricaria* (chamomile).

For premenstrual tension, use it with *Vitex agnus-castus* (chasteberry) and *Angelica sinensis* (Chinese angelica or dong quai).

For menopausal problems, try it with *Angelica sinensis* (Chinese angelica or dong quai), *Salvia officinalis* (sage) or *Leonurus cardiaca* (motherwort).

103

Capsules of evening primrose oil.

Panax ginseng (Korean ginseng)

Panax ginseng became a herbal superstar during the 1980s, when all sorts of claims were made for it, claims which tell us more about human hopes and dreams than they do about *Panax ginseng* itself. Especially if you were a man, it was said that it could make you dynamic, muscular, sexually potent and generally likely to succeed. Many people took it for a little while and were disappointed; others took too much and ended up being worse off than they were before; while some found that it worked for them.

After all of the hype, what's the truth about *Panax ginseng*? Like many plants, it contains substances that are very similar to human steroidal hormones. When you eat such plants, or take extracts of them, it is thought that they have two actions within the body. The first is to mimic the actions of human hormones, so that an extract of *Dioscorea villosa* (wild yam), which contains estrogen-like steroids, for example, can be used to prevent conception. The second is to act as a tonic for the hormone glands, helping them to regain their optimal functioning if they are not working well. Because the steroids within *Panax ginseng* resemble testosterone, they will have similar effects to testosterone: although they won't turn you into Superman or Superwoman, they will improve your stamina, energy levels and libido, but only if *Panax ginseng* is appropriate for you.

There are two groups of people for whom *Panax ginseng* can work wonders. The first consists of men and

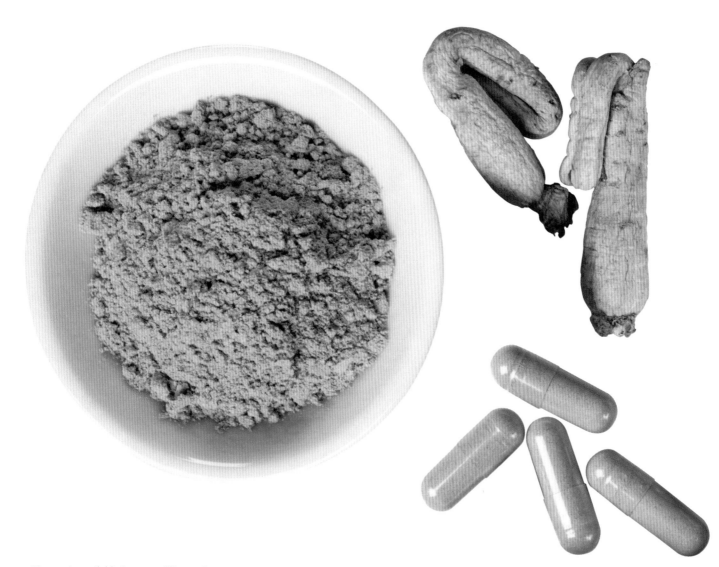

105

Ginseng is available in many different forms.

women who are basically well, but who feel that they need a boost for some reason – perhaps they have a race to run, an exam to pass, or just need a pick-me-up after a long, hard winter. If you take *Panax ginseng* for four to six weeks, it will give you a lift that will last for some months afterward. Take it for too long, however, and it will begin to deplete your vitality. Spring and autumn are good times to take *Panax ginseng*, when you may

need some help to sail through the change in season.

The second group consists of elderly people who feel that their life force has begun to diminish and who want to stay in good health for as long as possible. When taken continuously in old age, *Panax ginseng* helps to keep the home fires burning, easing the aches and pains of arthritis and supporting the functioning of the heart, liver and kidneys.

CAUTION !

Panax ginseng is not suitable for children or for women who are pregnant, trying to conceive, or nursing. Nor is it the right herb to take when you have an acute illness, such as a cold or a stomach upset. It is also too stimulating for people who are very debilitated, such as those suffering from myalgic encephalomyelitis (ME), who will need gentler, more nourishing remedies.

Plantago lanceolata (ribwort)

Remember the old wisdom about finding a dock leaf (*Rumex spp.*) with which to soothe the stings of nettles (*Urtica dioica*)? The leaves of *Plantago lanceolata* work just as well, and not only for nettle stings, but also for all kinds of cuts, stings and bites. If you rub a leaf between your hands, it will release some of its cooling, astringent juice, which you can apply directly to the affected area.

When taken internally, *Plantago lanceolata* offers the same kind of soothing, toning action to the stomach, throat and respiratory tract. It is excellent at drying up runny noses, but its special virtue comes into play in cases of allergic reaction, its anti-histaminic effect helping to head off the miserable symptoms of hay fever or any other mucus condition that may have an allergic component. Because it is very hard to avoid inhaling pollen and spores altogether, it is necessary to manage the allergic reactions that they may prompt. And, if the allergen is dietary, the most likely culprit is cows' milk and dairy products, so it's worth cutting these out of your diet for a week or so to see if that makes a difference. Such strategies, combined with taking *Plantago lanceolata* or other herbal mucus-membrane tonics, should really get to grips with the problem, and the improvement can sometimes be miraculous, particularly in small children who have been constantly sniffing.

Plantago lanceolata is gentle enough to be used to treat young children, yet strong enough to make a positive difference to hay fever (and sometimes asthma) sufferers of any age. It is even more effective when combined with herbs such as *Urtica dioica* (nettle) and *Euphrasia officinalis* (eyebright).

Rosmarinus officinalis (Rosemary)

Rosmarinus is a true tonic herb. Simply crushing and smelling a few leaves will act as a wake-up call to sleepyheads and students whose concentration is flagging. Its action is stimulating, bracing, focusing. It speeds up circulation and takes the edge off pain, making it useful particularly to headache sufferers and in pelvic inflammatory conditions. Rubbed into the scalp as a lotion or essential oil, it stimulates the hair follicles and can help hair to re-grow, or delay the progress of male pattern baldness.

It is harder to be depressed when taking Rosmarinus. It is a cheerful herb, steeped in sunshine, with a strong bitter element that acts on the liver as well as the head, cleansing and invigorating. If you are suffering from bitterness or jealousy, or have just become exhausted through caring too much, try inviting Rosmarinus into your life. Its traditional place as a companion to high-fat meats like lamb or mutton is no accident, either; it will counterbalance stodginess in food in the same way that it dispels heaviness of the spirit.

For depression, use it with *Verbena* (vervain), *Avena sativa* (oat straw), *Hypericum* (St. John's Wort) or *Borago officinalis* (borage or starflower). For headaches, try it with *Stachys betonica* (wood betony) or *Ginkgo biloba* (ginkgo). In treating pelvic problems of all sorts, Rosmarinus (rosemary) works well with *Glycyrrhiza* (licorice) and *Zingiber* (ginger), together with whatever herbs you are using for the particular condition.

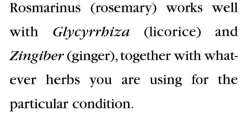

CAUTION !

Rosmarinus should not be used where there is high blood pressure, or by pregnant or breastfeeding women.

107

Rubus idaeus (raspberry leaf)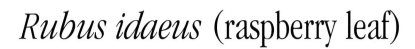

One use for *Rubus idaeus* has found its way into the mainstream: it is a uterine tonic, and women who drink the tea during the last three months of pregnancy are increasing their chance of having an efficient labor. Although I don't know of any systematic study of its actions (and it would be very difficult to do one), many midwives seem to have no doubts about its efficacy.

Rubus idaeus doesn't necessarily promise a short labor, but it can encourage an efficient one nevertheless. The walls of the womb contain three layers of muscle, whose fibers run in different directions: vertical, horizontal and diagonal. Each time a contraction occurs, these fibers shorten a little, until the cervix is pulled wide enough to allow the baby's head to pass through it. In a useful contraction, the muscles work together, moving with a wave-like action so that labor proceeds with the minimum amount of effort and pain. If there is tension within the muscles, however, perhaps because of the mother's anxiety or some physical reason, the muscle layers may pull against each other, resulting in painful contractions that do not help to dilate the cervix. This usually means a longer, and more difficult, labor.

The effect of *Rubus idaeus* is to improve the tone of the uterine muscles, thereby increasing the likelihood of labor proceeding smoothly. It can't help if the baby is presenting awkwardly or there is some other problem, of course, but it makes sense to prepare yourself as best you can for

108

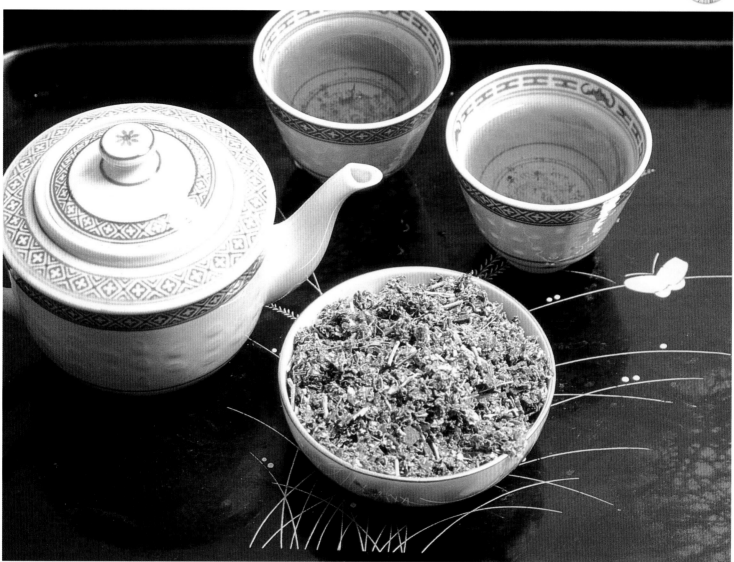

A cup of raspberry leaf tea can encourage a good labor.

labor, and *Rubus idaeus* can have a valuable part to play in this. Three months is long enough to take it, partly because you are likely to become bored with it if you keep drinking it for too long, and *Rubus idaeus* is not the most interesting-tasting tea! It is also a good idea to combine it with a herb like *Matricaria recutita* (chamomile) or *Melissa officinalis* (lemon balm), which will ease any digestive prob-lems that you may experience during the last weeks of pregnancy.

It may be useful to continue taking it for a few weeks following the birth because *Rubus idaeus* helps the womb to involute, or return to its nor-mal size, standing you in good stead for future pregnancies. This also helps to reduce the possibility of uterine prolapse in later life (and, indeed, it can be used to treat a prolapse if this does occur).

Rubus idaeus is a cheering, bracing kind of remedy, not showy or dramat-ic, but quietly efficient. Unobtrusive it may be, but its power should not be underestimated.

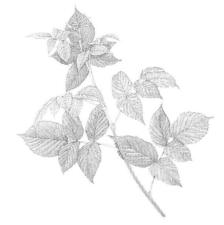

Salvia officinalis (sage)

Salvia officinalis is one of the many herbs used both in cooking and in medicine that originally grew in the Mediterranean area. Like its cousins, *Rosmarinus* (rosemary), *Thymus* (thyme) and *Origanum* (oregano and marjoram), among others, it carries within it the hot, dry quality of its native habitat.

Salvia officinalis also has some special qualities of its own. It is strongly antiseptic and also astringent, the two combined qualities making it an effective treatment for sore throats, in the form of a gargle (I have seen it clear up a sore throat almost instantly), and, as a mouthwash, for inflammation of the mouth and gums. The best way to prepare it is to boil a handful of leaves in 8fl. oz/250ml water for ten minutes and then to strain and cool the liquid before using it (be warned: it is very bitter.) It will keep in the fridge for up to twenty-four hours.

Another of the interesting properties of *Salvia officinalis* is that it reduces secretions of all kinds, from excessive salivation through heavy periods to the flow of breast milk (which can be useful when weaning a child) and sweating. This latter effect, combined with the fact that it has an estrogenic action, makes it an excellent remedy for hot flashes during menopause. It can effectively suppress night sweats, too, which are often a sign of debility, perhaps after a long period of illness. With its tonic effect and clarifying action, it is additionally a good herb for people who need to "pull themselves together."

Salvia officinalis combines well with *Glycyrrhiza glabra* (licorice) as a mouthwash and gargle.

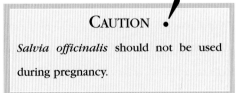

CAUTION !

Salvia officinalis should not be used during pregnancy.

Sambucus nigra (elder)

A fellow herbalist once went through all of the references to *Sambucus nigra* that she could find, counting the uses for it. There were forty-three in all – from repelling insects to protecting houses against lightning – making this herb a medicine chest in its own right. Its main use today is clearing phlegm from the upper respiratory tract. Warming and drying, *Sambucus nigra* encourages the flow of congested mucus and opens up blocked sinuses. It also helps to raise body temperature, encouraging the fever that often accompanies colds and flu to take hold, which in turn speeds up the immune response and enables the elimination of infection through sweating.

Any of its aerial parts can be used. The berries are rich in vitamin C, and when they ripen in early autumn you can make a cordial from them to use during the winter, when colds and sore throats threaten. Elderflower tea is one of the best herbal tisanes, one that even children will enjoy. Elderflowers lighten the spirit, as well as lifting congestion in the body, bringing fresh air into dark, stuffy places. Don't wait for a cold to try *Sambucus nigra*: its cheering, clearing powers will be welcome at any time.

Combined with *Achillea millefolium* (yarrow) and *Mentha piperita* (peppermint), *Sambucus nigra* is an excellent tea for colds, flu and sinus problems. To treat ear aches and infections, especially in children, try it with *Euphrasia officinalis* (eyebright), *Verbascum thapsus* (mullein) or *Echinacea spp.* (coneflower).

Symphytum officinale (comfrey)

FOR EXTERNAL
USE ONLY

If you look at a herbal guide that was written in times past, it will give you a very good insight into the kind of ailments that people once suffered from. Although we do not have many books dealing with the practice of medicine in Europe before those written by Nicholas Culpeper and his seventeenth-century contemporaries, these we do show that folk in those days were plagued by fevers, infectious diseases and wounds (mainly inflicted by each other). And by the time that written records began, *Symphytum officinale* was already firmly established as one of the best healers of wounds of all sorts.

Its magic ingredient is allantoin, a chemical that stimulates cells to reproduce faster and hence speeds up the repair of damaged tissues. Combine that with tannins, which help to draw the tissues together and form a protective seal, and lots of mucilage, which soothes and cools inflamed skin, and you can see why *Symphytum officinale* deserves its reputation. It works just as well whether the wound is external or internal: stomach ulcers and broken arms are all the same to *Symphytum officinale*. The one thing that it lacks, however, is the ability to discourage infection, so if that action is needed, you could combine it with a herb like *Calendula officinalis* (marigold) or *Echinacea angustifolia* or *purpurea* (coneflower).

Symphytum officinale gives solid support and nourishment on an emotional level, too, stabilizing and calming people in deep shock or pain due to, for example, bereavement, despair or serious illness. Its earthy quality also helps to ground and center a person who is having trouble keeping it together. Think of *Symphytum officinale* whenever direct physical action is needed: bandaging a wound, massaging a painful joint or giving a firm, heart-to-heart hug.

If you are dealing with an internal problem, such as a stomach ulcer, an irritable bowel or colitis, use the leaves for your preparation. The same applies if you take *Symphytum officinale* to soothe a persistent cough or to cool the ravages of arthritis. And if you are a vegan, note that the leaves of *Symphytum officinale* are one of the few plant sources of vitamin B12.

CAUTION !

Although they are wonderful when used in external preparations like creams, lotions and poultices, the roots of *Symphytum officinale* are not considered safe to eat.

Tanacetum parthenium (Feverfew)

Tanacetum parthenium is a powerhouse of a herb, containing over seventy active alkaloids. When you take it, it gets to work immediately, acting in two main ways. One is to calm down inflammatory arthritis, which was its best-known use until well into this century. The other is to open up the blood vessels, particularly in the head and neck – and this, of course, is the basis of its modern claim to fame as a treatment for migraine. Research has shown that when it is taken regularly over a period of three to four months at least, it helps about seventy percent of migraine sufferers.

That's very good news by any standards. But it's worth looking deeper when dealing with migraine. Although the bad headache is certainly partly caused by constricted blood vessels, and helping them to release will ease the pain, it is not the whole story. Migraine is a systemic disturbance, a cyclical storm that upsets stomachs – often to the point of vomiting – disturbs vision, and brings with it an "aura" of emotional malaise. For some sufferers, the headache is not the main feature of the migraine, and *Tanacetum parthenium* is unlikely to be of much help. In any case, it always pays to ask, why migraines? The answer usually lies in depletion of some sort: not eating well enough, taking too much out of yourself, or overburdening the liver in some way. Use herbs to treat the problem at a deeper level, and the migraines may, in time, disappear altogether.

Tanacetum parthenium can therefore be a useful top note in a prescription that might include *Verbena* (vervain), *Avena sativa* (oat straw), *Rosmarinus* (rosemary), *Stachys betonica* (wood betony), or *Taraxacum radix* (dandelion root). If you are taking Tanacetum parthenium on its own, rather than in a mixture, it is one of the few herbs that is best taken raw. The standard daily dosage would be five leaves, freshly picked or frozen, and it is a good idea to hide them in a sandwich, as they can cause irritation in the mouth. If you plant *Tanacetum parthenium* in your garden, you will always have a supply of fresh leaves, as it is difficult to get rid of, and seeds itself readily. Don't use leaves from the flowering stems, as these will have lost their potency.

For arthritis, it could be useful combined with *Glycyrrhiza* (licorice), *Apium graveolens* (celery seed), and some *Zingiber* (ginger).

113

Taraxacum officinale radix (dandelion root)

Taraxacum officinale is definitely a food rather than a medicine – in fact, the leaves are often used in salads and used to be grown in kitchen gardens for that purpose. Although the roots (T*araxacum officinale radix*) can be roasted and made into a coffee substitute, doing so is something of an insult to this herb. The only thing that it has in common with coffee is its bitterness; rather than giving you a quick buzz and upsetting your blood-sugar levels, it is solidly restorative.

Both the bitter taste of *Taraxacum officinale radix* and the constituents that give rise to the taste have a cleansing and stimulating effect on the liver, making it the first herb to choose to treat any problem to do with the liver or gall bladder. Illnesses that affect the liver, such as hepatitis or glandular fever, can leave a shadow months after the infection has passed, and *Taraxacum officinale radix* helps the liver finally to throw off the trouble. Likewise, if a person is, or has been, taking a course of drugs, it helps the liver to deal with the extra burden.

I see some people who have had their gall bladders removed, either because of digestive problems or because gallstones had developed. Although some feel fine after the operation, in others, the digestive symptoms – such as poor tolerance of fatty foods, gas, bloating, diarrhea or constipation – remain unchanged, if not worse than before. This is because gall-bladder trouble is a sign that something is wrong with the digestive system, and, because the gall bladder is not in itself the cause of the problem, removing the gall bladder will not necessarily solve it. In fact, without a gall bladder, the body can no longer control the release of bile into the small intestine, so that large, or

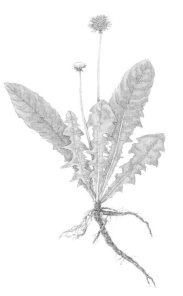

fatty, meals can be very difficult to digest. For such people, because it stimulates the release of bile from the liver and prepares the gut to cope with food, taking a small amount of *Taraxacum officinale radix* before a meal can avert hours of misery after.

The emotion that is traditionally associated with the liver is anger, and one symptom of a liver problem can be irritability or outbursts of temper.

Cooling and grounding, *Taraxacum officinale radix* will take the heat out of the situation, helping you to continue performing unrewarding tasks, such as caring for others, and will also allow you to retain a strong sense of self at times when you are feeling overwhelmed.

Taraxacum officinale radix combines well with *Matricaria* (chamomile) for treating digestive problems, and with *Echinacea* (coneflower) when an infection is involved.

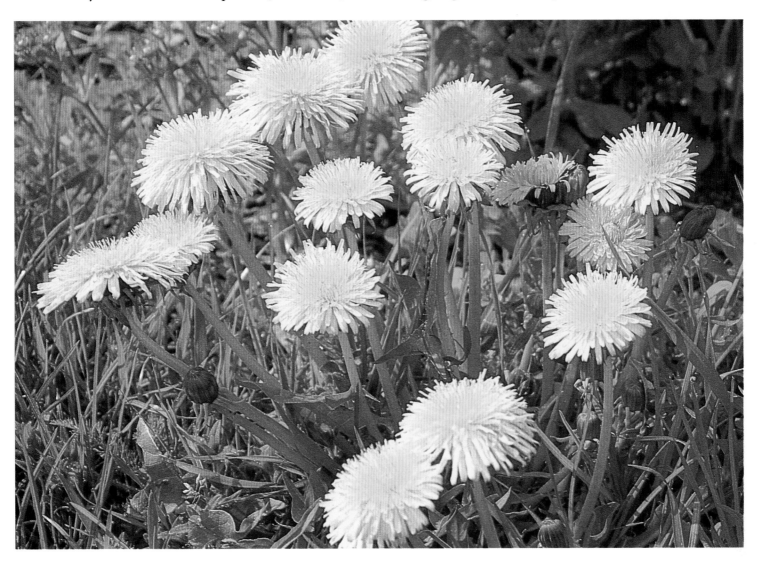

Thymus vulgaris (thyme)

Thymus vulgaris has been prized for centuries for the flavor that it bestows on food, especially meat and poultry. The oil that gives it much of its flavor yields other blessings, too. It calms spasms in the gut, for example, while stimulating the release of digestive juices, so that not only will you enjoy your chicken more when it is cooked with *Thymus vulgaris,* but you will digest it better. The oil is also a potent antiseptic, being active against bugs both within your food and within your body.

Like that of *Allium sativum* (garlic), its antiseptic action extends beyond the gut to other parts of the body, and it is especially useful for dealing with infections within the lungs, bronchi and sinuses, as well as the urinary system. *Thymus vulgaris* also spells death to fungal infections, such as athlete's foot. These can be very stubborn, however, but if you're persistent, constant applications of *Thymus vulgaris* cream – especially if you're also taking it as a tea or tincture – will eventually make the fungi so unhappy that they'll pack their bags and leave. But be warned: it's best to continue the treatment for a while after the symptoms have disappeared because fungal infections have a habit of going underground when times are hard, only to re-

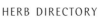

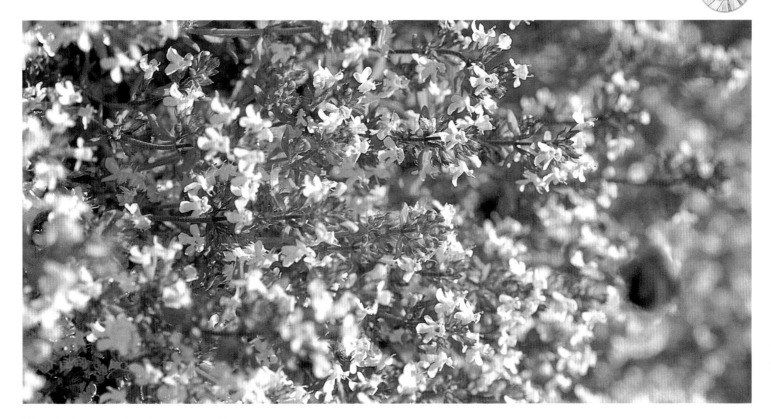

Thyme in flower, trapping the summer sunshine.

emerge when the coast is clear. *Thymus vulgaris* is one of the herbs that I use when treating thrush and other manifestations of candida.

The other main area of application for *Thymus vulgaris* is the respiratory system. It doesn't just combat infection, but also soothes spasms and irritation and promotes the flow of mucus, making it an excellent remedy for coughs, sinus problems, colds, sore throats and chest infections.

One of the beauties of *Thymus vulgaris* is that an ointment made with it can be rubbed onto the chest, enabling its volatile oil to diffuse into the lungs and bronchi (this is very useful when treating children who are reluctant to take medicine by

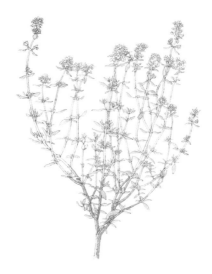

mouth). It works well as an inhalant, too. You can inhale it directly by adding a few drops of *Thymus vulgaris* oil to a bowl of very hot water and breathing in the steam so that it penetrate the sinuses and the upper respiratory tract. Or – and this is very

useful for treating children, along with anyone suffering from asthma or a persistent night cough – you can diffuse its active agents into the air by heating the oil in an essential oil burner.

Thymus vulgaris combines well with *Calendula* (marigold) and tea-tree oil as an effective cream or wash for treating fungal infections. For treating respiratory problems, it works well with *Echinacea* (coneflower) and *Plantago lanceolata* (ribwort). When the oil is used as an inhalant or a chest rub, it can be mixed with other oils, such as *Pinus sylvestris* (pine), *Mentha piperita* (peppermint) and *Eucalyptus globulus* (eucalyptus).

Tilia europea (lime flower)

Tilia europea is a gentle sedative that takes the edge off feelings of anxiety. It may be gentle, but it isn't weak, and a cup of *Tilia europea* tea will calm you down in minutes, as well as providing an effective nightcap for people who have trouble going to sleep. If you take it regularly, however, its action will move beyond that of a first-aid remedy and it will help to change patterns that are proving less than beneficial. When your response to stress has gone beyond rising to the occasion and you are suffering from the symptoms of anxiety, for example, it's time to seek the help of *Tilia europea.* In time, sleeplessness, and even panic attacks, will respond to its soothing touch, and it will also prove a good companion if you are coming off tranquilizers.

As you might expect, given its calming qualities, high blood pressure responds well to *Tilia europea.* Not only does it deal with the stress that can contribute to hypertension, but it works on hardened arteries, helping to dissolve away plaque and, if you build it into your daily routine, preventing further hardening. *Tilia europea*'s softening action works on hard hearts, too, extending an invitation to open up, relax and let the feelings flow. With its ability to embrace people who are frozen in grief, it offers the sense that it is safe to let go.

Tilia europea works well with *Crataegus* (hawthorn) and *Achillea* (yarrow) when treating high blood pressure. To alleviate panic attacks, try it with *Passiflora incarnata* (passion-flower) or *Leonurus cardiaca* (mother-wort). For coming off tranquilizers, combine it with *Carduus marianus* (blessed thistle) and *Passiflora incarnata* (passionflower).

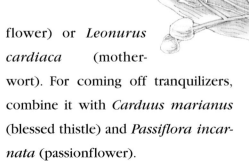

Urtica dioica (nettle)

As every gardener knows, nettles are strong and greedy, seizing any opportunity to invade disturbed ground and then dragging up nutrients from the soil and flourishing on their ill-gotten gains. In past times, folk knew how to claim back some of their stolen riches by collecting young and tender nettles in the spring, before crops of garden vegetables were ready to harvest.

As well as being rich in iron and vitamin C, *Urtica dioica* is generous with its vigor and acts as a metabolic stimulant, not in a depleting way like caffeine, but simply by waking up the system and making it move a little faster. Although this makes it the perfect spring tonic following the sluggishness of winter, it also helps people who are run down, anemic or recuperating from illness at any time of year. It will sharpen the appetite, too, while, paradoxically, aiding you if you are trying to lose weight (because of its stimulating and diuretic actions, Urtica dioica finds its way into many herbal slimming formulae).

This brings me to the reason why I have included *Urtica dioica* among the herbs that are good for the joints and muscles. It is a blood-cleanser, promoting the elimination of waste products from the body, particularly uric acid, which is implicated in inflammatory problems such as rheumatoid arthritis and gout. This also makes it useful in the treatment of chronic skin problems like eczema and persistent acne, along with fast-flaring conditions such as prickly heat and nettle rash.

Another of *Urtica dioica*'s virtues is its anti-histaminic action. As children quickly learn, if you touch its fresh leaves you will provoke a histaminic reaction in the form of a painful swelling. If you take a preparation of *Urtica dioica* internally, on the other hand, it will rapidly help to calm hay fever and other allergic responses. This quality may also play a part in how it takes the edge off rheumatic problems.

All of these qualities give *Urtica dioica* a strong claim as one of the most precious plants in the garden rather than a pest. In fact, it is a warrior, not a thief, and one that is willing to share its fighting spirit with us.

To alleviate gout and arthritis, take *Urtica dioica* with *Apium graveolens* (celery seed), *Glycyrrhiza glabra* (licorice), *Oenothera biennis* (evening primrose) or *Harpagophytum procumbens* (devil's claw).

For clearing up skin problems, try it with *Matricaria* (chamomile), *Calendula* (marigold) and *Rumex crispus* (curled dock).

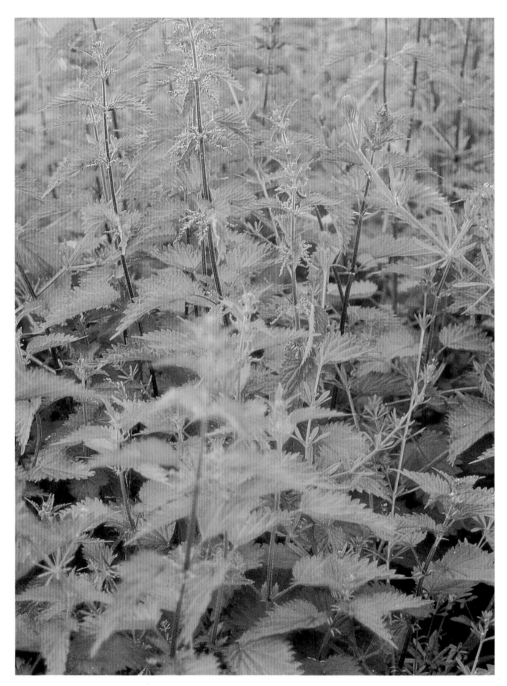

Nettle (*Urtica dioica*): full of strength and vigor.

To treat hay fever, combine *Urtica dioica* with *Plantago lanceolata* (ribwort) and *Euphrasia officinalis* (eyebright).

As a tonic, use it with *Verbena* (vervain), *Avena sativa* (oat straw) and *Galium aparine* (cleavers or goosegrass).

Valeriana officinalis (valerian)

Valeriana officinalis has one main virtue: it dispels anxiety, which makes it the mainstay of any mixture that is designed to target a problem in which anxiety plays a part, be it sleeplessness, panic attacks, palpitations or general "nerves." Because it is slightly sedative and takes the edge off pain, it can be useful when physical pain is causing stress. For countering the paralysis that is caused by fear, *Valeriana officinalis* is the first herb of choice, while it also acts a calming and reassuring friend if someone is suffering from the jitters that accompany the withdrawal from addictive substances.

In my experience, *Valeriana officinalis* works best if it is taken in short bursts, that is, for no more than about six weeks at a time.

(Caution: *Valeriana officinalis* can occasionally cause headaches (this is probably the body's response to its powerful smell). Another warning: don't leave it within reach of cats. Although it has a sedative effect on humans, it is highly stimulating to cats, so if they manage to eat some they'll go crazy for a while. Whether they, too, develop a headache afterward has, however, never been clearly established!)

121

Verbena officinalis (vervain)

Verbena officinalis is the herbal equivalent of chocolate, except that, instead of sweet seduction, it offers solid support. Grounding and centering, it gives you a firm place in which to stand, helping to establish a middle ground for anyone who is prone to mood swings, blood-sugar dips and cyclical problems like migraine. And the longer you take *Verbena officinalis,* the more problems you can deal with before being knocked off balance.

It is also very useful for people who are coming off any type of addictive substance, from drugs through alcohol and tobacco to sugar. Use it with cleansers like *Urtica* (nettle) and *Carduus marianus* (blessed thistle), as well as with calming herbs like *Hypericum* (St. John's Wort), *Valeriana* (valerian) or *Passiflora incarnata* (passionflower).

For alleviating migraines, *Verbena officinalis* works well with *Rosmarinus officinalis* (rosemary) and *Stachys betonica* (wood betony), and I have never had a patient who did not find some improvement after taking it. It is good for tension headaches, too.

For treating insomnia, try it with *Passiflora incarnata* (passionflower), *Humulus lupulus* (hop) or *Eschscholzia californica* (California poppy), to name but a few herbs.

For lifting depression, Verbena officinalis combines well with *Hypericum* (St. John's Wort), *Avena sativa* (oat straw), *Borago officinalis* (borage) or *Piper methysticum* (kava). It takes time for the full benefits to be felt, however, so don't give up if nothing seems to be changing during the first few weeks that of taking it.

To aid convalescence and recovery from stress of any sort, including serious illness, myalgic encephalomyelitis (ME), mononucleosis, bereavement and childbirth – anything that leaves you feeling depleted or debilitated – use *Verbena officinalis* with *Avena sativa* (oat straw), *Taraxacum officinale* (dandelion) and *Glycyrrhiza* (licorice).

122

CAUTION !

Verbena officinalis is best avoided during pregnancy.

Zea mays (corn silk)

Parts used: dried "silk" (stigmas and styles) of unripe corn.

Zea mays is a soothing remedy for inflammation in the urinary tract – a cup of Zea mays tea will ease the discomfort within twenty minutes (it doesn't taste bad, either, although it looks like horsehair). Its mildness makes it acceptable to children, and it is a useful remedy for bedwetting when combined with urinary astringents like *Equisetum arvense* (horsetail) and anxiety-reducers like *Matricaria recutita* (chamomile).

To treat cystitis and other infections of the urinary tract, use it with *Agropyron repens* (couch grass) and anti-infectives like *Echinacea* (coneflower) and *Thymus* (thyme).

Because it is strongly diuretic, once the irritation has died down, replace it with more astringent remedies like *Plantago lanceolata* (ribwort) or *Equisetum arvense* (horsetail).

123

Zingiber officinalis (ginger)

When using herbs like *Zingiber officinalis* and *Capsicum minimum* (cayenne) we are moving a step up from the warming herbs that are used both in cooking and in medicine. These two are downright hot, so much so that taking them can make you sweat. The obvious benefit of this effect is to cool you down, but it also aids elimination (a number of unwanted substances are excreted in sweat) and stimulates your circulation.

The usual dose of the tincture of *Zingiber officinalis* is very small: only two percent in 3fl. oz/100ml of other tinctures makes a week's worth of medicine. This is not enough to make you sweat, but sufficient to get the blood moving, right out to the capillaries in the hands and feet. It warms from the inside, too, stoking your internal fires so that you glow. *Zingiber officinalis* is, therefore, useful for treating all sorts of conditions where fire is needed, be it indigestion or arthritis, cold hands and feet or congestive pelvic problems like fibroids and pelvic inflammatory disease (PID). It can be used externally, too, to warm to sore joints and speed the healing of strains and sprains.

And because it boosts the circulation, if it is mixed with other herbs, it helps them reach the places where they are needed. *Zingiber officinalis* is a good companion herb, facilitating the work of others while doing a valuable job itself. Combining well with most herbs, you could think of it as the point of an arrow which adds drive to a remedy and ensures that it finds its mark.

124

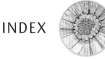

Index

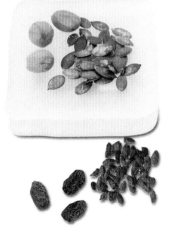
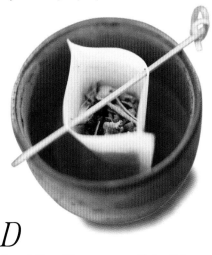

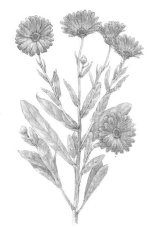

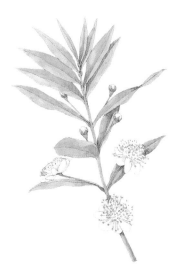

Acknowledgments

Thanks are due to Simon Mills and Christopher Hedley:
my first and best teachers.
Thanks also to my partner, Martin Wright, for his warm support
and constant optimism, and to my children, Rosie and Tom.

Picture Credits

Herb illustrations by David Ashby

© Photodisk: 1, 6bl, 7, 8tr, 9b, 11, 12br, 13, 15, 16br, 17, 18, 19, 20br, 21, 22, 25r, 26tr, 28br, 29tr, 32tl, 35, 36tr, 38b, 41tr, 47, 48bl, 49tr, 49br, 52b, 54tr, 55tr, 56b, 58bl, 58br, 59, 60tr, 63, 65tr, 68l, 69br, 70br, 71bl, 72tl, 73tl, 74, 75bl, 76br, 77, 79bl, 80bl, 81b, 82, 89, 103, 105, 109, 125

© Stockbyte: 9tr, 10bl, 10tr, 20tr, 24, 26b, 27, 29b, 30b, 33, 34b, 46tr, 48tr, 51b, 52t, 54br, 60br, 64bl, 67b, 69tl, 75tr, 78bl, 83

© McOnegal Botanical: 6tr, 8bl, 25l, 31, 36b, 50, 53, 55br, 57br, 6lb, 66b, 67l, 67tr, 70tl, 71br, 73br, 78tr, 94tl, 115b, 117t, 120

(t = top, b = bottom, l = left, r = right)

All other photography by Paul Forrester